How to Lose Weight Naturally

A Guide to Help Lose Weight, Be Healthy, and Reduce Your Risk of Disease

Take it off and keep it off!

By William J. Shuttic
CMT, CCN, CCH, CPT, CNHP

ISBN: 1511663987
ISBN 13: 9781511663984

Acknowledgements

I want to thank first and foremost my wife, Francie, who gave me moral support throughout this journey and stuck with me. I love you.

I also want to acknowledge my doctor friends and instructors including Robert Hudson LAc, Dr. Steve Schecter, Dr. Steven Ross, DC, FASBE, DAAPM, Jay Robb, and others, who taught me about anatomy and physiology, diet, exercise, and massage.

I want to thank all the doctors whose knowledge and information I have referenced for this book. Their dedication to the health and wellness of their patients is invaluable.

I want to thank my editors and art folks who helped put this book together.

And I want to give special thanks and appreciation to Dr. Steven Ross, who wrote the forward to this book.

Dedication

This book is dedicated to my father, William M. Shuttic, who has stood with me and supported me in all my endeavors throughout my life. I don't know of a more kind-hearted person than my father. Thank you for your support and love.

Forward

Obesity is an epidemic here in the United Sates, as well as in many other industrialized countries in the world. It is one of the leading causes of death, not because of the weight of the individual itself but, as a result of the progressive, degenerative diseases that it can and usually leads to. This was not the case 30 years ago but, with the change in our food sources, fast foods, "super-sized" meals not only in the fast food restaurants but in fine restaurants as well as our homes. It has become a necessity to super-size everything and everywhere from our food to our cars to our homes. Bigger is better.

The food industry has created foods that are "so delicious" that they become addictive. As a matter of fact, many of the ingredients and additives in processed foods today are on many of our genetic profiles as being addictive and intolerable. But, the Calvary has come to save the day (also known as Big Pharma). The pharmaceutical companies have followed-up by providing pharmaceutical answers to the symptoms, but not to the cause. As a result, we have become a nation of over-eaters and malnourished individuals leading to heart disease, diabetes, arthritis, dermatological inflammatory conditions, metabolic syndrome and so many more progressive degenerative disease that in fact, our life expectancy has decreased over the years, rather than increased as expected.

One of the key phrases we hear today in the health care community is...these are preventable and reversible diseases, if only we make the changes to our food intake, food consumption and instill a discipline of healthy nutrients, exercise and healthy hormones. Unfortunately, it sounds a lot easier than it really is. The internet is filled with quick fixes, the infomercials are ubiquitous, especially at night when you can't sleep due to your imbalance of nutrients and hormones. What is the truth, who do you believe, where should you spend my money? These are all very good questions and questions you should be asking before picking up the phone or your laptop to place your order. Much of what we see on television today as well as on the internet has little, if any real science behind them. So, who do you ask, where do you go? Well, if you have a practitioner who is well schooled in integrative or functional medicine that would be a good start. If you like to read science, you can always do your own research through such sites as www.pubmed.gov and type in the subject you are interested researching, and then sift through literally thousands of citations and papers on the subject. Or, you can read this book by an individual whom I have always respected and appreciated calling my friend and colleague.

I have known Bill Shuttic for over ten years. When I first moved to California from Minnesota in 2004 Bill was the first person I met in my office. He was a sales rep for a very reputable nutrition company at the time. He came in for a meeting to introduce himself and his company line and we struck up a friendship that has taken us both on various journeys. I have always found him very knowledgeable and always willing to help and research in the area of nutrition and overall health when I had questions posed by my patients. When Bill asked me to write the forward to his book, I was honored. "How to Lose Weight Naturally" is a terrific guide for not only those looking to lose weight but, for anyone wishing to expand their knowledge of nutrition, exercise, and bring back an overall healthy lifestyle. Bill takes complex subjects of health, wellness, biochemistry and physiology and puts them into easy to understand terms and easy to follow recommendations. Bill has "hit the nail on the head" with this book and I highly recommend this for everyone.

Don't get stuck in a rut because you are overwhelmed by all of the misinformation out there. Take some time for yourself and read, commit, study and work alongside Bill. You won't regret it.

Dr. Steven Ross

DC, FASBE, DAAPM
President and co-founder of The American College of Integrative and Functional Medicine (ACIFM) and President and CEO of Stellar Management Group

Table of Contents

Introduction

First of all, I'd like to thank you for buying this book. Secondly, I want to congratulate you for taking the first step toward becoming healthy and losing weight. I always like to say that just showing up is half the battle. You may have tried other weight loss programs or diets in the past. You may have gotten discouraged. But let me assure you that what I am going to show you is not a fad diet. It's a lifestyle. And if you can follow a few simple guidelines, it won't be long before you're looking and feeling great!

Before we get started, let me say that although I am certified as a Nutritionist, Herbalist, Massage Therapist, Personal Trainer, and Natural Health Care Professional, I am not a doctor. That being said, my education, I believe, is sufficient enough to give you the information you need to get you on your way to a healthy lifestyle. But in order to give my book more weight, I back up all of my opinions with information and comments from various doctors.

There is no one-size-fits-all. There is no magic pill. Everyone is unique. That being said, there are things that are common to good health. That's where we'll begin. From that point, you may have to do a little experimenting yourself to see what works best for you. In general, you'll need to exercise, you'll need to have a healthy diet, and you'll need to get enough rest. I'll go over some of the good things to do and some of the bad things not to do. I want to leave you with two things: the information you need to move forward with a healthy lifestyle and the means to get there. I hate when people tell me all the things I need to do but then don't give me a road map or any strategies or tactics to accomplish it.

At the end of this book, I've given you a starting point. I want you to write down your goals. How much do you weigh? How much do you want to weigh? How do you feel? How do you want to feel? What are your symptoms? Everyone is different. For me, when I hit two hundred pounds, that's when I knew it was time for me to get serious. Now I'm at a comfortable one hundred seventy pounds, and I'm pretty good with that. My body fat ranges from 15-18%. Where do you want to be? Do you want to be ripped and 9%? Write it down as one of your goals. If you've ever been heavy before, you'll know that it affects every part of your life. Psychologically, it may make you sad. It may lower your self-esteem. Physically, being heavy can drain your energy. You may feel slow both mentally and physically. You may have indigestion, bloating, headaches, etc. If you let it go on for too long, it could lead to diabetes, high blood pressure, digestive disorders, etc.

What you'll see is that being healthy really comes down to a few of things: diet, digestion, exercise, and keeping things in balance. Too much of anything will throw your system off. Too little of anything will throw your system off. This holds true for carbs, protein, fat, vitamins, minerals, exercise, etc. You'll also find that everyone has an opinion, and if you ask ten doctors their opinion on health or vitamins or whether you should be eating a high carb, high protein, or low fat diet, you may just get ten different opinions.

Along the same lines, the food you eat is extremely important. Is your food nutritious? Let me ask you, do you think a burger that you can buy for ninety-nine cents has any nutritional value? The food you eat gives you the nutrition to allow your body to function properly. Food that has no nutritional value has to be eliminated. If it is not eliminated, it will become toxic waste in your system which will get stored in your system and will lead not only to obesity but a host of other health issues.

Although this book is about weight loss, it is so important for you to understand that by changing your daily routine to a healthy lifestyle, not only will you lose weight, but you'll be reducing your risk of getting many chronic diseases such as diabetes, high blood pressure, high cholesterol, cancer, Crohn's Disease, Heart Disease, etc. I wrote this book with the hope that it will be able to answer some of the questions I had about weight loss, nutrition, and living healthy. I wish you the best in your journey to health.

Good Luck!

PS: Remember, losing weight will not make you healthy, but being healthy will help you lose weight.

COMMITMENT AGREEMENT

Commit to it! Don't Give Up!

I _____ am committed to changing my lifestyle to lead a more healthy and balanced life. I am committed to eating healthy. I am committed to losing weight. I know there will be good days and bad days, but I will not give up! I am committed to learning as much as I can about health and wellness. I will commit the next 90 days of my life to making the changes I need to be healthy.

_____

Signature

Take the 90-Day Challenge. Take a picture and/or video of yourself for the next 90 days and chronicle your transformation. Then you can post it for the world to see!

Chapter 1 – Why are we so fat?

According to the CDC:

Research has shown that as weight increases to reach the levels referred to as "overweight" and "obesity," the risks for the following conditions also increases:

- Coronary heart disease
- Type 2 diabetes
- Cancers (endometrial, breast, and colon)
- Hypertension (high blood pressure)
- Dyslipidemia (for example, high total cholesterol or high levels of triglycerides)
- Stroke
- Liver and Gallbladder disease
- Sleep apnea and respiratory problems
- Osteoarthritis (a degeneration of cartilage and its underlying bone within a joint)
- Gynecological problems (abnormal menses, infertility)

Also, according to Dr. Elson M. Haas, medical problems associated with obesity include:

Diabetes	Arthritis
High Cholesterol	Gout
Atherosclerosis	Varicose Veins
Hypertension	Gallbladder Disease
Heart Disease	Liver Disease
Kidney Disease	Menstrual Problems
Cancer	Infertility
Strokes	

(Staying Healthy with Nutrition, Elson M. Haas, p842)

It is important for you to live healthy and reduce your weight. It really can save your life. Although this book is about losing weight, I want you to understand that by losing weight, you are also increasing your health and decreasing your risk of disease. It is difficult for disease to live in a healthy body. Managing your weight is key to being healthy and happy. You should never be satisfied with poor health. So if you're sick and tired of being sick and tired, then now is the time to make the change.

A person with a Body Mass Index (BMI) between 25 and 29.9 is considered overweight. You would be considered obese if your BMI were over 30. According to the Center for Disease Control, the obesity rate in the United States currently stands at 35.7% of all adults, and 34% are overweight. That's almost 70% of people being either overweight or obese! Why is that? We spend the most money per capita on weight loss programs and healthcare. So, how is that possible? In my opinion, there are a number of reasons. First, of course, is that we have become a fast-food nation. We don't eat as much at home. Fast food is cheap and easy. We call that the SAD or Standard American Diet. Second, many kids today (and adults) don't get enough exercise. Thirty years ago, children would spend their time outside playing. Nowadays, kids sit at home playing video games. Lastly, the quality of the food we eat is just not that good. People don't eat a lot of fresh fruits and vegetables. We, as a nation, tend to eat processed food. Think about where you shop in the grocery store. How much time do you spend in the middle of the store buying pre-packaged and processed food? Here is a list of common food people buy:

The bread isle contains: white bread, whole wheat bread, multi-grain bread, seven-grain bread, rye bread, pumpernickel bread, sourdough bread, Italian bread, French bread, bread sticks, white bagels, raisin bagels, cheese bagels, garlic bagels, oat bread, flax bread, pita bread, dinner rolls, Kaiser rolls, poppy seed rolls, hamburger buns, hotdog buns.

Snack isle contains: crackers, pretzels, cookies, hoho's, ding dongs, candy, breakfast bars, chips.

Breakfast isle contains: cereals, waffle mix, pancake mix, syrup, Danish.

Baked goods isle contains: cake, pie, cookies, turnovers, scones, donuts, donut holes.

Pasta isle contains: spaghetti, lasagna, penne, elbows, shells, whole wheat pasta, green spinach pasta, orange tomato pasta, egg noodles, tiny-grained couscous, pasta sheets, Ramen.

Canned goods isle: processed fruits and vegetables and soups.

You are going to have to learn to wean yourself from these foods if you want to be healthy and lose weight. And yes, it is possible. You can either do it a little at a time or you can do it cold turkey. But if you want to lose weight, you need to start eliminating the foods that make you fat and unhealthy. You're going to have to re-educate yourself and learn an entirely new vocabulary with regard to health. Most importantly, you're going to have to learn to differentiate between what is good and bad for your health. And lastly, *you're going to have to do something about it!*

Processed Food

Why is processed food so bad? Processing food typically involves heating the food in order to sterilize it. Unfortunately, processing also kills all the good things that come in the raw form. When food is processed, it loses its enzymes. Enzymes play an important role in digesting food. Raw foods have their own enzymes. If you leave an apple out on the table, it doesn't take long before the enzymes begin to break down the apple. Although your body will produce its own enzymes, the enzymes in food aid in digestion.

Processing also removes vitamins and minerals from food. Therefore, you'll see labels that say, "fortified with 8 essential vitamins and minerals", and other similar things, because the natural vitamins have been removed and other vitamins and minerals (usually synthetic) have to be put back in.

Pesticides, Antibiotics, and Hormones

Another scary thing that happens in the food industry is the use of pesticides on crops and antibiotics and hormones on animals. Of course, if the animals are eating plants and grasses full of pesticides and have been pumped full of hormones and antibiotics, it's only logical that we are ingesting those things when we eat our steak or chicken. We are only beginning to discover the negative effects that has on our bodies. Pesticides are poison which will have a negative effect on your body. Antibiotics are over-prescribed in our society by doctors, so not only are we getting antibiotics from the food we eat but also directly from our medical establishment. An over-abundance or overuse of antibiotics will destroy the good bacteria in your gut and could lead to many health issues.

GMO's

There is also the discussion of genetically modified organisms or GMO's. On its face, GMO's may seem like a good idea. Crops that last longer and can survive where normal crops might fail. Science is a cool thing, but unfortunately, in the case of GMO's, messing with the genetics of our food supply may have an adverse effect on our bodies. Our bodies do not know how to breakdown GMO's, which can lead to a host of problems. Some people claim that the use of GMO's could lead to such things as Alzheimer's, ADHD, food sensitivities, allergies, inflammation, and more. I tend to agree.

There was a test done where animals were fed "Roundup Ready" beans which is a form of GMO. The results showed changes in the animals' liver, pancreatic tissue, intestinal tissue, and testicular tissue. There was a French study done in 2012 using GMO corn on rats, and the results showed that GMO corn caused cancerous tumors and killed seventy percent of female rats early.

There are books written about GMO's, so I won't go into it too much. Many countries have now banned GMO's. I would suggest avoiding GMO's and eating natural, organic, non-GMO foods.

Elizabeth Renter, a writer for NaturalSociety.com, has put together a list of the Top 10 Worst GMO Foods:

GMO Foods List: Top 10 Worst Foods

1. Corn

One of the most prominent GMO foods, avoiding corn is a no-brainer. If you've watched any food documentary, you know corn is highly modified. "As many as half of all U.S. farms growing corn for Monsanto are using genetically modified corn," and much of it is intended for human consumption. Monsanto's GMO corn has been tied to numerous health issues, including **weight gain and organ disruption.**

2. Soy

Found in tofu, vegetarian products, soybean oil, soy flour, and numerous other products, soy is also modified to resist herbicides. As of now, bio-tech giant Monsanto still has a tight grasp on the soybean market, with approximately 90 percent of soy being genetically engineered to resist Monsanto's herbicide Roundup. In one single year, 2006, there were 96.7 million pounds of glyphosate sprayed on soybeans alone.

3. Sugar

According to NaturalNews, genetically-modified sugar beets were introduced to the U.S. market in 2009. Like others, they've been modified by Monsanto to resist herbicides. Monsanto has even had USDA and court-related issues with the planting of its sugar beets, being ordered to remove seeds from the soil due to illegal approval.

4. Aspartame

Aspartame is a toxic additive used in numerous food products, and should be avoided for numerous reasons, including the fact that it is created with genetically modified bacteria.

5. Papayas

This one may come as a surprise to all of you tropical-fruit lovers. GMO papayas have been grown in Hawaii for consumption since 1999. Though they can't be sold to countries in the European Union, they are welcome with open arms in the U.S. and Canada.

6. Canola

One of the most chemically altered foods in the U.S. diet, canola oil is obtained from rapeseed through a series of chemical actions.

7. Cotton

Found in cotton oil, cotton originating in India and China in particular has serious risks.

8. Dairy

Your dairy products may contain growth hormones, since as many as one-fifth of all dairy cows in America are pumped with these hormones. In fact, Monsanto's health-hazardous rBGH has been banned in 27 countries, but is still in most US cows. If you must drink milk, buy organic.

9. and 10. Zucchini and Yellow Squash

Closely related, these two squash varieties are modified to resist viruses.

The dangers of some of these foods are well-known. The Bt toxin being used in GMO corn, for example, was recently detected in the blood of pregnant women and their babies. But perhaps more frightening are the risks that are still unknown. Even while these foods should be on your GMO foods list so that they are avoided, you can buy 100% organic to be safest.

Read more: http://naturalsociety.com/top-10-worst-gmo-foods-list/#ixzz306Zv1u6m

If you'd like more information on GMO's, I recommend watching a couple of videos and doing some research.

- GMO-OMG
- Genetic Roulette
- Food Matters

Chapter 2 - DIETS

My suggestion to losing weight is NOT to do a diet. (To lose weight, you need to lead a healthy lifestyle.) There have been many kinds of diets over the years. They typically don't work. Some may work while you're doing them, but as soon as you stop the diet, you gain the weight back. That is why it is so important to focus on being healthy, not on dieting to lose weight. Some of the various diets include:

The Atkins Diet. This is the original Low Carb Diet (in recent history, anyway.) It restricts your carb intake thus forcing your body into a state of ketosis using fat as fuel. It is very restrictive, and works only when you are on the diet. In the first phase, you are restricted to only 20 grams of carbs per day. That equals 80 calories. As soon as most people go back to eating carbs, they put the weight back on. Therefore, it has been classified as a fad diet.

The Mediterranean Diet. This diet has you eating a lot of fruits, veggies, beans, nuts, grains, fish, olive oil, with a little meat, dairy, and wine. It's good for your heart and so/so for weight loss. Some studies have shown that it may be better for weight loss than a low-fat diet. (You'll understand as you read further.)

The Blood Type Diet. This diet became popular with the book Eat Right 4 Your Type. It claims that people with different blood types have different needs, and by eating certain foods for your blood type, not only will you lose weight, but you'll be healthier, in general. You may want to look into it further.

The Paleo Diet. This is probably the most popular diet being promoted these days. It is also called the Caveman diet, because it is based on eating like our prehistoric ancestors of the Paleolithic Age. Because cavemen didn't farm, you can't eat sugar, dairy products, grains, or legumes. You can eat meat, fish, chicken, fruits, and veggies. This is also a low-carb diet, so you can lose weight. But can you go without eating carbs?

Raw Food. No cooking allowed. Everything you eat is in its raw form. The idea is that by cooking food, you kill the enzymes (true), therefore you don't digest properly. Proponents say that if you're eating cooked food, you're eating dead food with no value. You can lose weight on this diet, but it's another tough diet to follow. Raw foods are typically low in calories, fats, and sodium, and high in nutrients and fiber.

Macrobiotics. This diet favors organically grown, whole cereal grains (40-60%), followed by vegetables (20-30%), then sea vegetables (5-10%). A macrobiotic diet tends to avoid meat, animal fat, eggs, chicken, dairy, refined sugars, chocolate, honey, preservatives, refined foods, hot spices and alcohol.

Vegetarian. There are different levels of vegetarian diets. The Lacto-vegetarian does not eat meat, fish, chicken, or eggs, but dairy (milk, cheese, yogurt, butter, etc.) are OK. The Lacto-ovo vegetarian does not eat meat, chicken, or fish, but do eat dairy and eggs. The Ovo-vegetarian does not eat meat, chicken, fish, or dairy, but do eat eggs. You may find this surprising, but I have seen many fat vegetarians.

Vegan. Plant-based diet only. Vegans do not eat meat, fish, chicken, eggs, or dairy. Vegans need to pay special attention to make sure they get all their vitamins, minerals, and protein.

I'm not going to go through each diet in detail in this book. There's just too much to be said. I'll leave that for another time. Feel free to look them up and study each one. I also won't say any one diet is best for everyone. We are all different, and we all have our own separate needs.

The key to losing weight is simple – live a healthy lifestyle. What is a healthy lifestyle? It means putting certain things into your life and removing certain things from your life. I suggest you make a list of everything you do during your day. Then make two columns and write on the left side the things that are healthy and write on the right side the things that are unhealthy. For example:

Ate a grapefruit for breakfast	Had a donut for breakfast
Had a spinach salad for lunch	Had a bacon cheeseburger
Drank lemon water	Drank soda

If you have a second, stop reading this book for a minute and go grab a notebook. Call it your Health Journal or Wellness Notebook or something like that. You'll have better results if you write down and track your activities and your diet throughout the day. That way, you'll be able to see what's working and what's not. You'll also see when you haven't been as good as you thought you were.

Hippocrates, considered the father of medicine, said a couple of things that are very good to remember. He said, "Let your food be your medicine and your medicine be your food." He also said, "Whoever gives these things (food) no consideration, and is ignorant of them, how can he understand the diseases of man?" Smart guy!

Remember, one of the keys to losing weight and being really healthy is learning what foods are nutritious and what foods are harmful and how each affects you. So, the next thing we'll discuss is food information and labeling.

Chapter 3 – INFORMATION, EDUCATION, AND LABELING

Here's one problem – sometimes you don't know what is good and what is bad. There is so much information out there. Who knows what to believe? That's why I'm writing this book. What I learned becoming a nutritionist and herbalist was often different than what was being promoted on TV or even by doctors. Keep this in mind – in science and health, things are constantly changing, and sometimes what is written in stone today is disproved 5-10 years later. Don't believe me? Remember when fake eggs were supposed to be better than real eggs? Remember when fake sugar was considered healthy? Margarine was touted as being better than butter. Diet soda better than regular soda? In the future, I think we'll look back on some of the things we consider healthy today and say, "what were we thinking?" For example, radiation and chemotherapy treatment for cancer, I believe, will soon be thought of as barbaric. In the end, we'll have to go back to natural food. Also, doctors get very little training in nutrition, which I find very surprising. Thankfully, many doctors nowadays are beginning to get trained as Naturopathic Doctors. I highly suggest you seek out a Naturopath to discuss your health goals with.

Since the 1980's the health industry has been telling us that fat is bad, so we should be eating a low-fat diet. So, we've been told to eat more grain and less fat. Low-fat, fat-free, etc. has been the mantra. In that same period, our country has become the most obese country in the world. According to the CDC, there was a dramatic increase in obesity from 1990 through 2010.

"In 1990, among states participating in the Behavioral Risk Factor Surveillance System, 10 states had a prevalence of obesity less than 10% and no state had prevalence equal to or greater than 15%. By 2000, no state had a prevalence of obesity less than 10%, 23 states had a prevalence between 20 – 24%, and no state had prevalence equal to or greater than 25%. In 2010, no state had a prevalence of obesity less than 20%. Thirty-six states had a prevalence equal to or greater than 25%; 12 of these states (Alabama, Arkansas, Kentucky, Louisiana, Michigan, Mississippi, Missouri, Oklahoma, South Carolina, Tennessee, Texas, and West Virginia) had a prevalence equal to or greater than 30%."

When I was studying nutrition, we learned all of the benefits of fat on the body. Fat is so important to so many aspects of your physiology that most people have no idea about. Of course, there are healthy and unhealthy fats. Here are some of the positive effects of fat:

- Fat is necessary for certain fat-soluble vitamins to work

- Fat insulates your body

- Your brain needs fat

We'll discuss fats in greater detail later.

Labeling

Another thing you need to know is the facts behind the label. Following is an excerpt from an excellent article at www.projectswole.com:

Some examples of "healthy food" words on product labels:

- *Fat Free*

- *Reduced Fat*

- *Low Fat*

- *Sugar Free*

- *No Added Sugar*

- *Diet*

We are supposed to believe that each of these categories makes a food healthier. In reality, this couldn't be further from the truth.

Here is what those "healthy food" phrases actually translate to:

- *Fat free, but full of sugar and chemicals.*

- *Reduced fat, but increased carbohydrates.*

- *Low fat, but high glycemic index..*

- *Sugar free, but artificial everything else.*

- *No added sugar... because the all-natural version has enough sugar to give you type II diabetes anyway.*

- *"Diet" food, but it causes cancer in lab rats so don't drink/eat too much of it.*

Consider the logic that food manufactures would have us believe: fat-free is good for you; jelly beans, jolly ranchers, and cotton candy are fat-free; therefore all those sugary candies are good for you. Makes sense? Think about it.

In fact, a study at John Hopkins University recently determined a link between high blood sugar and heart disease. This means high glycemic foods, such as the candy I just mentioned as well as many similar products, are inherently unhealthy.

Here is a list of how sugar is labeled. You need to be aware of this, because if you see any of these on the label, you're ingesting sugar.

Barley malt	Corn syrup solids
Fruit juice	Honey
Beet sugar	Date sugar
Fruit juice concentrate	Maltodextrin
Invert sugar	Brown sugar
Dextran	Glucose
Lactose	Buttered syrup
Dextrose	Glucose solids
Malt syrup	Cane-juice crystals
Diatase	Golden sugar

(www.thealternativedaily.com)

Here's another thing about labeling you may not know. If your food has a little label stuck on it, it will probably have a number on it. That number can tell you a lot about the food you're eating. Let's take an apple, for example. Next time you're at the store, look at the label on the apples. Most likely, it will have a number like 4123. The "4" means that it is conventionally grown. That's sounds pretty good, right? But conventionally grown means that it may have been grown with the use of chemical pesticides, herbicides, or fertilizers, could be GMO or could have been irradiated. If your apple is organic, it will have a "9" before the "4". A GMO food might have an "8" before the "4". So, you can see the importance of knowing what is on your label.

With regard to vitamins, there are natural vitamins and synthetic vitamins. Any Naturopath will tell you that the natural vitamins are better than the synthetic vitamins. Whenever you see a study done on vitamins, see which type of vitamins they were testing. If the results say that vitamins are bad, the vitamins tested were probably synthetic. How do you know the difference? Let me give you an example. The scientific term for one of the E vitamins is d-alpha tocopherol. The "d" represents a right-spinning molecule. Some vitamins have a prefix of "L" which represents a left-spinning molecule. A natural vitamin cannot have both the "d" and the "L" prefix. Yet you will often see something with a "dl" prefix. Only a synthetically-made vitamin can be "dl". You should avoid vitamins that are "dl".

There is a lot of misinformation out there. According to Infinity's Complete Physique:

"...heart disease – the number one killer today – has been blamed on "dietary saturated fat and cholesterol." Recently, Consumers' Research magazine said this is a "health scam," and that heart disease is "not what you think." Instead, heart disease is linked to "devitalized" or "fabricated" foods, including refined sugar, pasteurized milk, soft drinks, fortified white flour, imitation broth products, egg powders and even synthetic vitamins."

14

They also said that:

"...the American Dietetic Association is largely funded by trade groups and food companies. The article says the ADA takes the "wishy-washy stance" that there are not "good or bad foods," because they rely on industry money which "means that they never criticize the food industry."

Let's review some common foods and drinks and test your education and information.

Wheat/Gluten – good or bad?

There is now more science coming out showing that a diet high in whole grains/gluten may not be as healthy as we once thought. (Gluten is a protein within wheat.) Here are some of the downsides of eating too many grains:

Refined grains, which are carbs, break down quickly in the system, spike blood sugar levels, and create an insulin response. The excess glucose in the blood is then converted to fat.

Here are two reasons why wheat may not be good for us. First, if you're a believer in the Paleo Diet (see above), some believe that man today is essentially the same as we were a hundred thousand years ago. And way back then, people ate nuts and berries and animal protein. Farming didn't come for many thousands of years later. So the theory goes that man was never really meant to eat grain. It's a valid theory, but I'm not sure I buy it completely. The second reason, which I find more compelling is that the wheat we eat today has been hybridized into a dwarf wheat that has different properties from the wheat grown fifty to one hundred years ago. A geneticist named Norman Borlaug developed the dwarf wheat, and he even won a Nobel Peace Prize for it. On the good side, it did help increase crop yields which is good for world hunger. On the downside, this is another example of where man thinks he can create something better than nature/God. Even though I love new technology, I tend to lean toward nature over man.

I highly recommend reading Wheat Belly by Dr. William Davis, M.D. He is a cardiologist who has seen people lose 20-50 pounds within a few months simply by removing wheat from their diets. Of course, that flies in the face of the current point of view from the medical community and the FDA. According to Dr. Davis:

"A wheat belly represents the accumulation of fat that results from years of consuming foods that trigger insulin, the hormone of fat storage. While some people store fat in their buttocks and thighs, most people collect ungainly fat around the middle. This "central" or "visceral" fat is unique: Unlike fat in other body areas, it provokes inflammatory phenomena, distorts insulin responses, and issues abnormal metabolic signals to the rest of the body. In the unwitting wheat-bellied male, visceral fat also produces estrogen, creating "man breasts"."

There was also a Mayo Clinic study done in conjunction with the University of Iowa that studied 215 obese patients. Their study showed that a wheat-free diet in these patients resulted in 27.5 pounds weight lost over a six month period.

The next question is, "I was told eating whole grains was good for me. If I cut out the grain, maybe I'll lose weight, but will I be healthy?" According to Dr. Davis:

"Documented peculiar effects of wheat on humans include appetite stimulation, exposure to brain-active exorphins (the counterpart of internally derived endorphins), exaggerated blood sugar surges that trigger cycles of satiety alternating with heightened appetite, the process of glycation that underlies disease and aging, inflammatory and pH effects that erode cartilage and damage bone, and activation of disordered immune responses. A complex range of diseases results from consumption of wheat, from celiac disease – the devastating intestinal disease that develops from exposure to wheat gluten – to an assortment of neurological disorders, diabetes,

heart disease, arthritis, curious rashes, and the paralyzing delusions of schizophrenia."

When I learned that, I was shocked. But it makes sense. Some people are overweight because they drink too many sodas and eat burgers and fries all day long. But I know people who don't eat junk food, they exercise regularly, they eat a low-fat diet, they watch their calories, they eat healthy whole wheat, and yet they're still fat! Are you one of those people?

MILK

I know doctors and the media continue to tell you to drink your milk. You've probably heard it since you were a child. But what makes milk good for you? Or is it even good for you at all? Typically, the reason you're told to drink milk is because of the protein content and Vitamin D. So, you drink milk to get protein. Since our society is on a low-fat fad, we're supposed to drink that watered-down, low-fat, or no-fat milk. I don't know about you, but I think low fat milk is pretty nasty. Now, back in the day, raw milk was good for you. It came with all the good bacteria and enzymes that would help to digest the milk. Nowadays, milk is highly processed. As I mentioned earlier, the processing uses heat and removes most of the nutrients from the milk. So what you're drinking now is more like a watered down protein drink. The enzyme that breaks down the lactose in milk is called lactase. Our bodies only produce lactase as children and decreases as we get older. Have you ever wondered why so many people are lactose intolerant? It's because they either don't produce lactase or produce very little, so they can't digest the milk. Milk causes inflammation and mucus within your body. A glass of milk contains 135 million pus cells, bovine growth hormone, antibiotics, 51 milligrams of cholesterol, 300 calories, 16 grams of fat, and acidic protein which leeches calcium from bones.

In my opinion, I don't think adults should be drinking milk in their daily diets. Let me tell you a little secret. I usually have a cup of coffee every morning. I don't put milk in my coffee. I put cream in my coffee. Heavy cream. That's right. And even consuming heavy cream, I was able to lose 20 pounds. That kind of makes you go hmmmmm...

There is a huge difference between raw milk and today's processed milk. Raw milk, being natural, is good for you. Processed milk...not so much. But today's laws are making it more difficult to buy raw milk, which is really unfortunate. Following is an excellent article from NaturalNews.com:

Raw Milk Vs. Processed Milk

A complete protein – Raw milk contains all 22 amino acids, including the eight essential amino acids needed for the complete metabolism and function of protein. This makes raw milk a perfect protein source, and especially good for growing children and bodybuilders. The proteins in processed milk, however, don't fare as well. The milk's biological value is reduced by 17 percent because the heating process damages at least two of these amino acids (lysine and histidine). Moreover, this damage to the amino acids' identity negatively affects their absorption rate in the body.

Rich in vitamins – Raw milk is rich in fat-soluble vitamins A, D, E, K as well as B and C– the entire vitamin spectrum. It is a particularly potent B vitamin complex, with all the major B vitamins, from biotin to B12, represented. In treated milk, though, vitamins A and C are completely destroyed (infants fed pasteurized milk exclusively actually develop scurvy), while pasteurization destroys approximately 38 percent of the milk's all-important B vitamins. Vitamins D, E, and K appear to survive the heating process.

Healthy fats – Raw milk contains all 18 fatty acids (saturated and unsaturated) that are metabolically available to us, including conjugated linoleic acid, a much-needed omega-6 fatty acid. These fats – which our bodies cannot make themselves – aid cellular metabolism, the formation of healthy cell membranes, brain and endocrine system function, and much more. Processed milk, on the other hand, is a different story. While pasteurization is bad enough (it compromises the milk's fat content), homogenization – a truly unnatural process that presses milk fats into smaller globules – actually oxidizes these fats, making them carcinogenic and toxic to the body.

Bursting with enzymes – Raw milk contains over 60 known enzymes that perform a multitude of tasks in our bodies. Some of these enzymes, such as lipase, are native to milk and help us digest it properly. Other enzymes, such as catalase, lysozyme, and lactoperoxidase, help protect the milk from bacterial infections. In treated milk, many of these enzymes are completely destroyed, including lipase – the very enzyme needed to digest milk properly.

Rich in minerals – Raw milk contains a large number of metabolically-available minerals. Some of these are well-known macro-minerals such as calcium, magnesium, and phosphorus, whereas others are important trace minerals such as iodine. Since minerals work in tandem rather than in isolation, disrupting the mineral compositions of whole foods such as milk can lead to numerous problems. And can you guess what happens to treated milk? Yes; having had its precious minerals compromised by aggressive heating and pressing treatments, the milk becomes toxic. Its total amount of soluble calcium is especially affected, and since phosphorus and magnesium need calcium to function properly (and vice versa), you can see how this nutritional instability can cause a chain reaction of problems in our bodies.

High in beneficial cholesterol and carbohydrates – Raw milk contains about 3 milligrams of cholesterol (an important repair substance) per gram, as well as decent amounts of soluble carbohydrates. The primary carbohydrate in cow's milk is lactose, which makes up approximately 2-8 percent of milk by weight. Individuals with lactose tolerance cannot make this enzyme, and thus cannot digest milk sugar. However, since raw milk (unlike treated milk) retains its lactose-digesting Lactobacilli bacteria, people with lactose intolerance often have no problems drinking it. (Michael Ravensthorpe, Natural News)

Diet Soda

This is another one of those things that I believe will soon be changing. In fact, I believe it's already changing. Remember when diet soda was supposed to be better than regular soda because it has zero calories and replaces sugar with artificial sweeteners? Well, how's that working out for you? Do you drink diet soda? Has it caused you to lose any weight? As it turns out, we're beginning to find out that artificial sweeteners and coloring in diet sodas not only is carcinogenic and can cause cancer, but it also makes you crave sweets. This means you are either drinking more diet sodas or eating more processed sugars, fats, and carbs. It's time to ditch the sodas – both regular and diet – and switch over to something healthier.

Here are some of the negative effects of diet soda:

- The phosphoric acid weakens your bones and teeth
- Artificial sweeteners make you crave more
- The coloring has no value other than adding color and is carcinogenic
- Aspartame will break down into formaldehyde in your system
- High fructose corn syrup can increase body fat, cholesterol, and triglycerides
- Potassium benzoate will break down into benzene which is carcinogenic
- Food dyes can impair brain function and has been implicated in ADHD

High Protein/Low Carb

Popularized in the 80's with the Atkins Diet, this is also another diet that may be a little unbalanced. I believe their diet has been adjusted recently, so I won't bash the Atkins Diet too much, but a diet that is too high in protein and too low in carbs is unhealthy. This is how Felicia Drury Kliment puts it:

"...if the objective in losing weight is to improve health, that should be the driving force behind the choice of diet. The high-protein, low carbohydrate diet does not fulfill that objective because it is unbalanced. Eating so little starch deprives the body of glucose, its primary source of fuel, while eating too much meat threatens the body's mineral reserves. Excessive phosphate levels in meat can remove calcium and magnesium in the teeth and bones. Another danger to the body's supply of alkaline minerals is blood nitrogen urea from the breakdown of meat. Too much meat in the diet produces excessively high urea levels that the kidneys excrete along with magnesium and calcium."

The loss of calcium from a high-protein/low carb diet may lead to osteoporosis.

Also, a diet that has excessive protein and almost no carbs has a negative effect on your kidneys. When your body doesn't have enough carbs, your body will burn ketones from fat metabolism. With a continued lack of carbs; ketosis will occur which raises the amount of acid in your blood. That acid is processed by the kidneys. With time, the kidneys become overworked and damaged, and you run the risk of getting kidney stones. Some people promote ketosis for weight loss, but you should be aware of the risks.

High Carb/Low Fat

A high carb, low fat diet is also unbalanced and has a double whammy. The carbs will create an insulin response, so your blood sugar will first spike and then drop. The carbs will be converted to fat. A high carb diet will lead to obesity. Not enough fat in your diet has a number of effects on your body. Fat makes you feel full. Without fat, you may feel hungry all the time. Also, in order to get your calories, the missing fat calories will be made up with carb calories. Keep in mind, also, that many of the vitamins you eat are fat soluble and need fat in order to be used. Without fat, your vitamins may not be working.

Here's what some people do, unfortunately. They go on a high carb/low fat diet and they reduce their caloric intake. They even exercise. When they don't lose weight, they can't figure it out, so they cut back even further on fat and cut back even further on calories. Yet they still can't lose weight. They're doing exactly the opposite of what they should be doing! In fact, when you do this, you are decreasing your metabolism, making it even more difficult to lose weight. Are you one of those people? Fat and protein are both necessary for your body's health and also to lose weight.

There are some doctors who will tell you that you should be eating 50-60% carbs. One of those doctors is Elson Haas, MD. Dr. Haas is actually one of my favorite doctors. His books should be on your reading list. In my opinion, the only way I would recommend a 60% carb diet is if all those carbs were vegetables. I prefer something closer to the 40/30/30 rule.

Coffee

I'm sure by now you won't be surprised when I tell you that coffee can be both good and bad. Recently, green coffee beans were being touted by people such as Dr. Oz as a great weight loss supplement. Coffee increases your metabolism and that makes it effective as a weight-loss agent. Of course, it could also increase your blood pressure. Coffee is also acidic and if you add sugar, additionally so. So, as with most things, a little coffee is not a bad thing, but too much is not healthy. The most recent study that came out said that up to five cups of coffee per day is ok. That seems a little high to me. I'd try to keep my limit to three cups.

Salt

A discussion is needed about salt. Doctors typically tell you to cut down on your salt intake in order to reduce cholesterol, high blood pressure, etc. It's not necessarily that salt that is hurting you, but rather the form of the salt. Table salt is sodium chloride (NaCl). As it turns out, sodium is not bad for you, but sodium chloride is. Your body needs a certain amount of organic sodium. Sodium is one of the body's main electrolytes. Sodium chloride, however, cannot be used by the body. It cannot be used for our metabolism because sodium chloride comes from rocks as opposed to organic sodium which comes from plants. There have been clinical studies that prove this:

"One study revealed that when sodium chloride was given to individuals who are prone to hypertension, their blood pressure rose, but when organic sodium was given to these same people, their blood pressure moved towards normal. It was also found that sodium chloride induced the body to lose calcium, whereas organic sodium induced a decrease in calcium loss. An interesting fact arose in this study that completely baffled the researchers. Whenever sodium chloride was ingested, the body quickly removed it. However, when organic sodium was given, the body held it."

(Cleanse and Purify Thyself, Richard Anderson, ND, p. 27)

Organic sodium is needed for many things in the body, one of which is balancing the body's pH. I will discuss pH later in this book. My suggestion would be to throw out your table salt and try using Himalayan salt or some type of sea salt.

Chapter 4 – Macro Nutrients: Carbs, Fat, Protein

Carbs, Protein, and Fat - Good vs. Bad

Over the years, some people have tried to put carbs, protein, and fat into one of two categories – good or bad. Some say carbs are good, fat is bad. Some say the opposite. Who is correct? Well, as it turns out, there are good and bad carbs, good and bad fats, and protein can be both good and bad. Well, that really complicates things, doesn't it?

First, let's talk about **calories**.

1 gram Fat = 9 calories

1 gram Carbs = 4 calories

1 gram Protein = 4 calories

So, if you're counting calories, you would think it makes sense to eat less fat. BUT…is counting calories the right thing to do? Counting calories goes back to the old thinking of "calories in, calories out," but here's the problem with that (and feel free to test this out yourself.) If you base everything on calories, then it wouldn't matter if you ate 2,000 calories of Pop-Tarts and Oreos or 2,000 calories of chicken or vegetables. My point is that it's not the calories but the *calorie to nutrient ratio*. Your body uses nutrients to stay healthy and heal itself. The nutrients you eat have an effect on your metabolism, and your body self-adjusts (your body is pretty smart) depending on what nutrients are present or not. So if you'd like to test it out, eat 2,000 calories of junk food for a month and see how things go at the gym and see what happens to your body. Then, eat 2,000 calories of fruits and vegetables only and see what happens.

This is not a new concept that I discovered (I wish I could claim credit for it.) According to Luis Balart, MD and Sam Andrews, MD who wrote the #1 bestseller Sugar Busters say:

"Research has shown that, as we diet and lose weight, the body changes the amount of energy it expends. The body adjusts its energy requirements downward and thus needs to expend less energy to run itself [Leibel, Rosenbaum, and Hirsch, 1995]. This presents a form of resistance to maintaining a reduced weight even while maintaining exactly the same low-calorie diet. This startling phenomenon accounts for the poor long-term results of most dietary treatments of obesity."

(Sugar Busters, Balart, Andrews, Bethea, & Steward, p. 30)

The point is that it's not the calories that count but the nutrients. We've been sold a bill of goods by the diet industry. Learn the truth. Change your habits. Be healthy.

Getting back to good vs. bad carbs, protein, and fat...

Let's start with carbs.

When somebody mentions carbs to you, what do you think? Take a second. I ask this because so many times I hear people talking about carbs but they fail to differentiate between good carbs and bad carbs. So we really need to begin by defining the different types of carbs, so as not to be confused. Carbs provide the main source of energy for your body. There are simple carbs and complex carbs.

Technically, carbs can be broken down into monosaccharides, disaccharides, and polysaccharides (saccharide = carb). Monosaccharides are the simplest carb and act as quick fuel for the body. Some examples include galactose, fructose, and glucose. Disaccharides are sometimes referred to as simple carbohydrates. These are the carbs that we tend to eat a lot of in processed form. Processed fruit juice, white rice, white flour, cereal, and candy are examples of disaccharides. Polysaccharides are the complex carbohydrates that typically have fiber in them. This allows them to break down more slowly and scrub your intestines. Whole grains, brown rice, and vegetables are examples of complex carbs.

Good carbs are unrefined. Good carbs include fresh fruits and vegetables. Healthy carb sources are high in fiber, so looking at the fiber content on the Nutrition Facts label is a great way to identify them. A high-fiber food contains at least 5 grams of fiber per serving. Bad carbs are anything refined and most of the things you're probably buying at the grocery store. If it comes in a box and sits on the shelf, it's probably not a good carb. I know it seems kind of weird to think that broccoli is a carb and a donut is a carb. But big difference. That's why it is important to differentiate between good and bad carbs.

Carrots are considered carbs. One cup of carrots contains about 50 calories, very little fat, but a lot of vitamins, minerals, and enzymes. A slice of wheat bread contains about 69 calories, 1 gram of fat, a small amount of calcium and iron, but not much in the way of vitamins or enzymes.

According to Livestrong.com, a glazed donut contains about 240 calories and 120 of those calories are from (saturated) fat. A large donut could have as many as 327 calories. Donuts are also made with hydrogenated oils which is doubly bad.

An overabundance of bad carbs leads to obesity. Remember, carbs are a food source that get broken down into simple sugar. Conversely, a prolonged deficiency in good carbs will cause a breakdown of protein (and muscle), a loss of energy, and an imbalance in electrolytes (sodium and potassium). Carbs help build bones and skin tissue and it helps lubricate joints. The good carbs that have fiber are good for keeping your colon clean. I will discuss sugar and fiber later in this book.

It is very possible to get addicted to the "bad carbs" because they tend to make you feel good in the short term. Why? When you eat carbs, it causes an insulin reaction. That, in turn, causes the amino acid tryptophan to reach the brain. Your brain then turns that into serotonin which makes you feel good and makes you sleepy. So, one of the key ways to lose weight is to wean yourself off of the "bad" carbs. That has both a mental component and a physical component. If you're motivated enough, the mental part is easy. The more difficult part of breaking your carb addiction is the physical part. Sugar can be as addictive as cocaine, and when you stop eating it, you will get withdrawals. My friend Jay Robb wrote a book called the Fat Burning Diet. In it, he says:

"All 'mental' carbohydrate addictions can be broken in one thought. Most 'physical' carbohydrate addictions are broken in a matter of four days, which is the amount of time required for insulin levels to stabilize and also for the body to eliminate most traces of the offending carbohydrate based foods. This includes breaking most allergy addictions to heavy carbohydrates (such as sugar, corn syrup, and all sweet foods), as well as common staples (such as wheat, potatoes, oats, corn, rye, barley and other starchy grains.)"

(The Fat Burning Diet, Jay Robb, p38)

Fat. Same question here as applies to carbs. When someone says fat, what kind of food comes to mind? There are different kinds of fat. Some are good for you. Others are not so good. I'm going to forego the discussion on long-chain vs. short-chain molecular structure. I won't bore you with the chemistry. Fat does combine with carbon to form triglycerides which plays a role in your health and disease. Fats are important in the transportation and absorption of certain vitamins such as Vitamins A, D, E, and K. These are called fat-soluble vitamins. We will cover water-soluble vitamins in the Vitamin Section.

There are various types of fats – some good and some bad. Let's briefly go through the different types of fats and what makes them good or bad. There are saturated fats, unsaturated fats, hydrogenated fats, and the EFA's.

Good Fats:

Monounsaturated Fats - Omega 9

Polyunsaturated Fats – Omega 3 and Omega 6 (Essential Fatty Acids)

Bad Fats:

Trans Fats (Hydrogenated)

Saturated Fats

Saturated and Trans Fats

Trans Fats are oils that have been "saturated" with hydrogen in a man-made process that keeps the oil from spoiling. Margarine is a good example of a hydrogenated trans fat. These oils were once thought to be healthy, but we now know that trans fats raise your LDL cholesterol levels, lower your HDL cholesterol, and increase the risk of cardiovascular disease. I consider trans fats kind of a Franken-oil. It's another example, in my opinion, of a man-made product not being as good as a natural product.

Saturated fats are normally found in animals. They harden up at room temperature. Saturated fats are better to cook with because they are more stable and take longer to go rancid. You can find saturated fats in beef, pork, lamb, chicken, milk, butter, cheese, coconut oil, and yogurt. Saturated fats are typically considered the "bad" fats, but coconut oil, as it turns out, is very healthy and good for you.

Saturated fats can raise your LDL (bad cholesterol), may lower HDL (good cholesterol) and increase your risk of heart disease and stroke.

A recent study has come out that says that dietary fat does not affect your blood cholesterol levels. This may have a dramatic impact on the way your doctor talks to you about your health.

Trans fats and saturated fats are found in such things as donuts, French fries, pastries, biscuits, pizza, as well as margarine and fat-replacement shortenings.

EFAs

There are essential fatty acids which we need but can't be produced in the body. According to Dr. D. Rudin, only 20% of our needs are available in the average diet today.

There are two types of essential fatty acids (EFA): Omega-3 and Omega 6. Omega-3's are more reactive than Omega-6's. They both play an important role in health but for different reasons. Omega-3's promote growth, keeps the skin supple, and supports the integrity of cell membranes.

EFAs are converted into prostaglandins which help regulate the entire body. Without EFAs, your digestion will not work efficiently and your body's healing capacity is compromised. According to Dr. David F. Horrobin, the following conditions have been helped by Gamma linolenic acid (an Omega 6):

"Alcoholism, atopic eczema, breast pain, cancer, cardiovascular disease, diabetic neuropathy, endometriosis, gastrointestinal disorders, liver disease, post-viral fatigue syndrome, PMS, renal disease, rheumatoid arthritis and other forms of inflammation, schizophrenia, and dry eyes." (Putting It All Together p. 79.)

For EFAs to work well, your body needs to have certain nutrients. Ascorbic acid, biotin, calcium, magnesium, pyridoxine, zinc, and B3 allow EFAs to do their job effectively. (This is one reason you may want to take vitamins. We'll discuss vitamins later.)

The other Omega fatty acid is the Omega 9. It is a monounsaturated fat that you get from food. The main Omega 9 fatty acid is Oleic acid. It is found in canola, olive, and sunflower oil. Omega 9 can be found in fruits, nuts, and oils.

U.S. Food and Drug Administration recently approved a Qualified Health Claim for canola oil saying,

"limited and not conclusive scientific evidence suggests that eating about 1½ tablespoons (19 grams) of canola oil daily may reduce the risk of coronary heart disease due to the unsaturated fat content in canola oil. To achieve this possible benefit, canola oil is to replace a similar amount of saturated fat and not increase the total number of calories you eat in a day." (www.omega-9oils.com)

The interesting thing about that is that many Naturopaths will avoid canola oil because it is a GMO and has been genetically modified. This is a perfect example of how natural health professionals have differing opinions from the mainstream medical industry and our own government.

Will you get fat by eating fat? That is the million dollar question. The answer is yes and no. According to Dr. Hoffer (and other doctors) food fat by itself will not cause heart disease, does not elevate blood fats, and will not make you fat. How does he come to that conclusion? Because there are people throughout the world who eat high levels of fat who don't get fat and don't get heart disease. The Somalis and Samburus' diet is about 2/3 saturated fat, yet they have a low level of heart disease. Also, I've seen people who do the Atkins diet lose weight while eating large amounts of fat. So what's the key? As mentioned above, fats need other nutrients to work effectively. Second, if fat is combined with sugar (ie. Ice cream, donuts), it is basically fat, white flour, and sucrose and becomes the ultimate processed food poison. People then get addicted to the sweet taste and overeat. And sugar will deplete the vitamins in your system. The second key is fiber. The less fiber you have, the higher your blood fat content.

Heat breaks down fat, so cold pressed oils are typically better. When heat breaks down oil, the oil becomes rancid which is bad for your system.

Unsaturated fats can be mono-unsaturated or poly-unsaturated. To keep from spoiling, these fats should be stored in a dark bottle and kept in a cool, dry place or refrigerated.

> Monounsaturated fat – examples include Olive Oil, Canola Oil, and Almond Oil

> Polyunsaturated fat – examples include Soybean Oil, Safflower Oil, Sunflower oil, Cottonseed Oil, Corn Oil, Sesame Oil, Peanut Oil.

Essential Fatty Acids – EFAs: (also called Vitamin F). EFAs are all poly-unsaturated oils.

> Omega 3 – Also called Linolenic Acid. Examples include Flax-seed Oil, Soybean Oil, Canola Oil, Pumpkin Oil, Walnut Oil, and cold-water Fish Oil.

> Omega 6 – Also called Linoleic Acid. Examples include Soybean Oil, Safflower Oil, Sunflower Oil, Corn Oil, Wheat Germ Oil, and Sesame Oil.

Let me explain why you need fat. Fat serves as an energy source for the body. There are 4,000 calories per pound of fat. Fats add flavor to food which allows you to enjoy your food. (Have you noticed that many diet foods taste terrible?) Fat gives you your curves! We all want to have some curves, right? Of course, we don't want to let that get out of control. Fat builds a protective sheath around nerves and other organs for protection. And, of course, fat serves as an insulator that will keep you warm. Good fats help improve cholesterol levels, reduce the risk of heart disease, reduce the risk of diabetes, improves vitamin absorption, promotes cell development, and is needed for a healthy immune system.

When you go shopping, you can find good fats in avocados, olives, almonds, pistachios, walnuts, salmon, and tuna.

What is interesting to note are certain trends in this country. A poor diet leads to both obesity and diabetes. Diabetes is an epidemic. But look at the statistics. According to Dr. Steward,

"The rate of diabetes in the United States has more than tripled since 1958, which correlates closely with the increased amount of sugar consumption...The percentage of fat consumed per person since the late 1970's has actually decreased from 40 percent to 33 percent, and more important, the actual consumption in grams per person per day is down from 85 grams to 73 grams (a 16 percent drop). Yet the incidence of obesity has doubled since the late 1970's and people weigh eleven to twelve pounds more than when they were consuming larger quantities of fat!"(Sugar Busters, p. 85)

Good Fats	Bad Fats
Monounsaturated (Omega-9) Liquid at room temperature and naturally occur in many foods	**Trans** Most are artificially produced as a result of partial hydrogenation, which is a process used to convert liquid oil to a solid
Polyunsaturated (Omega-3, Omega-6) Liquid at room temperature and naturally occur in many foods	**Saturated** Typically solid at room temperature and naturally occur in foods such as meat

(www.goodfats101.com)

The last word on fats. Some authorities are beginning to question whether saturated fat is really bad for your health. As mentioned, coconut oil has incredible health properties. For the time being, I suggest staying away from saturated fat until more information is available. As for vegetable oil, you may want to avoid canola oil, cottonseed oil, safflower oil, and soybean oil due to them being GMO.

Lastly, let's discuss protein.

Protein is made up of amino acids. There are twenty-two naturally occurring amino acids. Amino means "nitrogen containing" which means that nitrogen is essential to our health. There are essential and non-essential amino acids.

Essential Amino Acids

- Valine
- Methionine
- Tryptophan
- Threonine
- Phenylalanine
- Lysine
- Leucine
- Isoleucine

Non-Essential Amino Acids

- Serine
- Glycine
- Glutamic Acid
- Aspartic Acid
- Asparagine
- Alanine

Conditionally-Essential Amino Acids

- Tyrosine
- Taurine
- Proline
- Glutamine

- Cysteine
- Arginine
- Histidine

Essential amino acids we need to get from food, as our bodies do not produce them. Protein makes up about 20% of your body's composition (as compared to 60% for water.) Protein makes up a part of your muscles, hair, nails, skin, eyes, heart, and brain. When we discuss exercise, we'll go over how protein builds muscle which helps burn more calories which leads to weight loss. Your body breaks down an average of 300mg of protein per day. Many doctors claim that you only need 50-60 grams of protein daily. If you spend a lot of time working out in the gym and are actively trying to gain muscle mass, you may need more. A personal trainer might suggest taking 1-2 grams of protein per pound of body weight. For a 180 pound man, that would mean 180-360 grams. The RDA only recommends 0.36 grams of protein per pound of body weight. I recently read that a 200 pound man should take 200 grams of protein taken as 40 grams per meal with five meals per day. Amino acids are essential for both weight loss and health. Most amino acids are utilized to make enzymes, hormones, antibodies, and muscle.

People have asked me if eating too much protein can cause fat. The answer is yes, it can. It can be stored in the body as fat or stored as glycogen in the liver. Not enough protein, on the other hand, can cause weight loss due to muscle breakdown and other health issues. (When we lose weight, we want to lose fat, not muscle.) Normally, when your body needs energy, it will burn carbs first, fat second, and protein last (unless you're starving; then your body holds fat.) Also, protein will give you a longer, slower energy burn and not spike your blood sugar like carbs will.

Proteins help maintain sodium/potassium balance in the body and helps normalize your body's acid/base balance. Protein is also needed to produce hydrochloric acid which your body needs in the digestion process. It helps heal wounds, regulates hormones, and produces antibodies. Without protein, you may have difficulty losing weight, you could have cold hands and feet, and you could have food cravings. Another question I hear often is, "when should I eat protein?" I would suggest eating your protein for breakfast and after working out. If you eat carbs for breakfast, your blood sugar will spike, you'll get an insulin response, your blood sugar will drop, and you'll be hungry in a couple hours. That means you may want to switch from oatmeal to a veggie omelet in the morning.

In the end, obesity is caused more often from an over-consumption of processed carbohydrates than too much protein or fat.

Portions and proportions

I've seen some doctors recommend only 10% of your diet should be composed of fat. Other doctors say that carbs should comprise 10% of your diet. Who is right?! Personally, I go with the 40/30/30 plan. 40% carbs, 30% protein, and 30% fat. Of course, those are the good carbs and the good fats. Remember, if you are spending a lot of time in the gym, some people will take 1 gram of protein per pound of body weight. That may be excessive for some people. If you're just an average guy or girl working 9-5 and not spending much time at the gym, you may only need 50-60 grams of protein per day. A general rule of thumb would be that you need to get at least 30% of your body weight in protein (measured in grams).

If you're more of a B-Type and you don't want to count the grams or the calories, a simple rule of thumb would be that when you eat, your protein should be about the size of your open hand, and your carbs should be about the size of your closed fist. Think of a chicken fillet and a small lump of rice. I make an exception with vegetables. I think that half of your meal could be in the form of vegetables.

Good sources of protein (and amino acids) include:

- Pumpkin seeds
- Almonds
- Sunflower seeds
- Walnuts
- Tempeh
- Brazil nuts
- Pistachios
- Legumes
- Animal products (but some people don't like eating animal protein. Your choice)

Chapter 5 – Micro Nutrients: Vitamins and Minerals

Are vitamins really necessary? Are they really good or a waste of money? That seems to be a never-ending question that never dies. Personally, I think vitamins are a good thing, and I believe everyone should be taking at least a multivitamin daily. But you'll hear some doctors constantly saying how vitamins are bad for you, or vitamins are worthless, or vitamins are dangerous, etc. Some people make the claim that because vitamins are not regulated by the FDA, you have to be careful. Personally, I don't want the FDA anywhere near my vitamins. I don't want the government telling me I have to get a prescription for my vitamin C! Of course, there will be good quality and bad quality vitamins, just like anything else. If you're paying less than $20 for a month supply of vitamins, you're probably buying some pretty cheap stuff. You know the old saying, "you get what you pay for." I suggest doing a little research on different brands of vitamins. The two brands I use are either from Beach Body or Jay Robb. But I'm sure there are other good brands on the market. Try to find Whole Food Vitamins. Look for vegetarian capsules if you go for the capsule vitamins.

When you hear about vitamins going straight through people and ending up in the toilet, it could be due to a number of reasons. First, you could be taking low quality pills that aren't digesting in your system. Another reason may be that your digestive system is simply not working efficiently and isn't breaking the vitamins down in your system. (This is why I always recommend doing a cleanse first, as well as taking enzymes and enough fat.)

The next question is how much do you need? That gets us into information and labeling. Most of us probably go back to the old RDA – Recommended Daily Allowance – to find out how much of each vitamin we need. Unfortunately, that's probably not the best place to go. The **Recommended Dietary Allowance** or **RDA** (sometimes referred to as *Recommended Daily Allowance*) is defined as "the average daily dietary intake level that is sufficient to meet the nutrient requirements of nearly all (approximately 98 percent) healthy individuals."

I want you to notice that the RDA is the recommended amount for healthy individuals. Think about that. If you think you're okay because you've reached your RDA, you may want to rethink that. If you are overweight; if you have health issues; if you have high cholesterol, high blood pressure, acid reflux, indigestion, headaches, joint pain, etc. you probably need more than the RDA suggests. Sometimes much more. For example, I believe the RDA for Vitamin C is 60 milligrams. I know people, myself included, who have taken 6,000 milligrams of Vitamin C per day. Huge difference. The other thing to consider is your size and if you are male or female. Do you think a 100 pound woman has the same requirements as a 200 pound man? Do you think a sickly person has the same requirements as an athlete? More recently, the government has adopted something called the DRI or Dietary Reference Intakes to provide the recommended daily allowance of nutrients. According to the Department of Agriculture website:

"So the Board (Food and Nutrition Board of the National Academy of Sciences) replaced and expanded the current RDAs with Dietary Reference Intakes (DRIs) to provide recommended nutrient intakes for use in a variety of settings. The DRIs are actually a set of four reference values.

Recommended Dietary Allowance (RDA) is the average daily dietary intake of a nutrient that is sufficient to meet the requirement of nearly all (97-98%) healthy persons.

Adequate Intake (AI) for a nutrient is similar to the ESADDI and is only established when an RDA cannot be determined. Therefore a nutrient either has an RDA or an AI. The AI is based on observed intakes of the nutrient by a group of healthy persons.

Tolerable Upper Intake Level (UL) is the highest daily intake of a nutrient that is likely to pose no risks of toxicity for almost all individuals. As intake above the UL increases, risk increases.

Estimated Average Requirement (EAR) is the amount of a nutrient that is estimated to meet the requirement of half of all healthy individuals in the population.

Each of these reference values distinguishes between gender and different life stages. RDAs, AIs and ULs are dietary guidelines for individuals, whereas EARs provide guidelines for groups and populations. In addition, factors that might modify these guidelines, such as bio-availability of nutrients from different sources, nutrient-nutrient and nutrient-drug interactions, and intakes from food fortificants and supplements, are incorporated into the guidelines in much greater detail than previously."

(http://www.ars.usda.gov/News/docs.htm?docid=10870)

What that means is that as time progresses, we're learning that the old RDA was underestimating the amount of vitamins that we need. This also allows me to get back on my soap box and repeat that things are constantly changing, and what is true today may not be true tomorrow. Naturopaths have been saying for years that mega-vitamin supplementation may not only be good for us, but may also help cure certain ailments.

There are doctors nowadays that use vitamins not only as prevention but to treat conditions. Vitamins have been used over the past hundred years to treat both physical and mental ailments.

Vitamins work together in harmony as a symphony. They need each other. I am a firm believer in something called Orthomolecular nutrition which is basically using either mega-doses or optimal doses of vitamins and minerals for specific issues.

There are water-soluble vitamins and fat-soluble vitamins. Water soluble vitamins will be excreted if you take too much, so there's not really any concern about taking too much. Fat-soluble vitamins need fat to be effective. It is possible to ingest too much fat-soluble vitamins.

I'm a huge proponent of Vitamin C. I suggest reading the works of Dr. Linus Pauling to get more information. He used mega-doses of Vitamin C to cure many diseases. In 1990, at a meeting in Maryland sponsored by the National Cancer Institute, they came to the following conclusions regarding Vitamin C and the treatment of cancer:

1. *Ascorbic Acid (Vit C) protected plasma lipids against oxidative damage...*

2. *Ascorbic acid decreased the toxicity against normal tissue of drugs used in chemotherapy and decreased the toxicity of radiation, but it did not protect the cancer.*

3. *Ascorbic acid had anticancer properties...*

4. *...33 out of 46 studies vitamin C was protective, decreasing cancer incidence and mortality.*

5. *Ascorbic acid had properties that make it an important part of any cancer treatment.*

(p170 – Putting It All Together)

Vitamins can increase your metabolism, provide energy, reduce cravings, and suppress your appetite.

Vitamins

Vitamin A (Fat Soluble)

Vitamin A is an anti-oxidant, anti-infective, and anti-carcinogenic vitamin that is vital in the development of skin, bone, lung tissue, teeth, mucous membranes, urinary tract, intestinal tract, and epithelial tissue. It can be converted into retinol which is a nutrient used for night vision and color. Vitamin A can help prevent osteoporosis by allowing for the uptake of phosphate and sulfate. It is needed for the synthesis of sex hormones. It keeps the digestive tract healthy thus guarding against ulcers. Did you know Vitamin A did all that? Vitamin A can be depleted by pollution and the processing of food which removes vitamins. Alcohol also depletes Vitamin A from your liver. Vitamin A can be found in animal sources: liver, butter, whole milk, cheese, egg yolk, and vegetables: spinach, beet greens, carrots, and turnips. If you do not have enough Vitamin A in your system, you may get frequent infections, have brittle nails, cloudy vision, brittle nails, itchy dry eyes, dry and brittle hair, dry skin, and skin rashes.

Vitamin B (Water-soluble)

In general, the B-Vitamins are taken together as a B-Complex. They have the ability to unlock the fuel in carbs, fats, and proteins. As a whole, B-Vitamins work with enzymes to release energy from the food and supplements you ingest. B-Vitamins play a key role in the metabolism of carbs, fats, and protein and helps normalize your digestion and appetite. They help fight fatigue by supplying the body with oxygen. B-Vitamins are used in Detox programs because they can help detox the liver and protects against cardiovascular disease. They help with your nervous system by allowing your enzymes to produce neurotransmitters which could be useful for schizophrenia, psychosis, and depression. B-Vitamins can be depleted by alcohol, coffee, tea, and stress.

B-Vitamins	Male DRI	Female DRI
B1 = Thiamin	1.4mg	1.0mg
B2 = Riboflavin	1.6mg	1.2mg
B3 = Niacin	18mg	13mg
B5 = Pantothenic Acid		
B6 = Pyroxidine	2.0mg	2.0mg
B12 = Cobolamine	3.0mg	3.0mg
Folic Acid	400mcg	400mcg

B1 – Thiamin – functions in carb metabolism and helps nerve cells. It facilitates the movement of potassium and sodium back and forth across the nerve cell membranes in the body. B1 is also a co-factor for acetyl choline which is a neurotransmitter that helps your body create energy. It also helps keep the muscle tone of your digestive tract strong and firm, allowing for good digestion and elimination. A lack of B1 could cause nerve disorders, mental problems, cardiac problems, and can change your mood and mental state. On a mild level, a B1 deficiency could cause a burning sensation in the feet, depression, poor circulation, headaches, insomnia, and indigestion. A severe deficiency could cause edema, an enlarged heart and liver, heart palpitations, weak muscles, and breathing difficulties. Much of your B1 can be lost by cooking or boiling food, so of course, raw is better. B1 can be found in yeast, whole grains, liver, pork, and legumes. Although the RDA is 1-1.4mg/day, some Naturopaths will recommend 15-20mg/day. There is currently a B-Vitamin product on the market that has 300mg of B1.

B2 – Riboflavin – is also used in carb metabolism. It helps with the breakdown of fats and is needed for activation of folate and Vitamin B6. B2 also works within the glandular system. It causes the pituitary gland to secrete ACTH (a hormone) which, in turn, causes the adrenal glands to secrete hormones which help regulate the sodium/potassium balance, which help to lower blood pressure. Vitamin B2 can be found in yeast, dairy, liver, meat, eggs, fish, walnuts, dark green veggies, nuts, beans, grains, tofu, tempeh, and miso. Vegans are often deficient in B2. Alcohol, baking soda, and antibiotics also block the absorption of B2. RDA is 1-1.6mg/day, but like B1, some recommend 15-20mg/day.

B3 – Niacin – was discovered in 1937. There are two types of Niacin – nicotinic acid and nicotinomide. Both are naturally found in foods. Niacin is made from the amino acid tryptophan with the help of Vitamin B6. Taking niacin can cause flushing of your skin, but that is not a bad thing. Personally, I like it, but some people don't like the heat. Niacin is useful for fat metabolism but it has also been used for people with osteo-arthritis, high cholesterol, migraines, cold hands and feet, atherosclerosis, and Bells Paulsy. It can lower LDL cholesterol and raise HDL. It is a vaso-dilator. Niacin can be toxic if you consume too much. The RDA is 14-16mg/day, but some Naturopaths will recommend 50mg/day.

B5 – Pantothenic Acid – was discovered in 1939 and functions in fat, carb, and steroid metabolism. B5 is concentrated in your adrenal glands. It converts carbs, fats, and protein into energy as well as acting as an anti-stress agent. Your adrenals synthesize cortisol, which is a steroid hormone. B5 is useful for allergies, insomnia, and inflammatory conditions. It can be found in liver, organ meats, brewer's yeast, grains, legumes, nuts, seeds, veggies, fruits, and animal products. Too much stress, low blood sugar, and allergies can deplete B5.

B6 – Pyridoxine – has more functions than any other B Vitamin. B6 acts primarily as a Co-Enzyme and helps enzymes involved with amino acid synthesis, breakdown, and conversion. For example, B6 allows tryptophan to create serotonin and niacin; B6 allows tyrosine to produce dopamine and nor-epinephrine; B6 allows lysine to produce carnitine; and B6 allows homo-cysteine to produce cysteine which produces the anti-oxidant, glutathione. (Homocysteine is related to heart disease and B6 can help reduce homocysteine levels in your blood.) B6 allows amino acids to create energy; B6 is needed for metabolism of essential fatty acids; B6 is necessary for the formation of hemoglobin; B6 is needed to get glycogen (stored carbs) out of storage; and B6 breaks down estrogen in the liver. Processing food removes a lot of B6, and you can see how important it is. Pregnant women, women on oral contraceptives, and people concerned with cancer should all be sure to get enough B6. A lack of B6 could lead to depression, poor muscle function, and stiff joints. Things that interfere with B6 include: alcohol, birth control pills, asthma medication, cortisone, prednisone, toxins, tobacco. B6 has been used for PMS, carpal tunnel syndrome, iron-resistant anemia, heart disease, kidney stones, and asthma. RDA for B6 is 1.2-1.7mg/day, but some Naturopaths will recommend 35-50mg/day. B6 can be found in bananas and pears, brown rice, salmon and herring, liver, and brewer's yeast.

B12 – Cobalamin – was discovered in 1948 as people were then trying to deal with pernicious anemia. Anemia is caused by a lack of B12 and Folate, not by an iron deficiency, as was once thought. B12 is an extremely complex molecule. B12 is the only water-soluble molecule that the body stores. People typically take B12 pills or shots when they are feeling tired or fatigued. There are various types of B12 including cyanacobalamin (synthetic), methylcobalamin (a food form which is active in the body), adenosylcobalamin (a food form which is active in the body), and hydroxocobalamin (a food form which is not active in the body.) Check your vitamins to see which form of B12 is being used. I believe most use cyanacobalamin, which is the synthetic form and not as good as the natural form. In order for B12 to be absorbed, it must interact with Intrinsic Factor which carries B12 across the cell wall in the intestines into the blood stream. B12 is heavily stored in the liver. B12 converts homocysteine to methionine and activates Folic Acid which builds DNA. Pharmaceuticals that block acid production in the stomach (Zantac, Tagamet, etc.) stop not only HCL production but also stops Intrinsic Factor, too. Remember, Intrinsic Factor is needed for B12 absorption. B12 is important for the health of your gastrointestinal tract, bone marrow, blood, liver, nervous and metabolic systems. RDA for B12 is 2.4mcg/day, but some Naturopaths recommend 25-50mcg/day up to as much as 1000mcg/day.

Folate – Folic Acid – was discovered in the 1940's. Folate helps in the synthesis of DNA and also reduces homocysteine levels in the blood. Pregnant women, in particular, need to be aware of their folate levels, because a deficiency could lead to pregnancy issues. Folate is minimized by aspirin, birth control pills, sulfa drugs, diuretics, and alcohol. Vitamin C increases the absorbability of folate. Folate can be found in chicken liver, organ meats, egg yolks, spinach, broccoli, mushrooms, legumes, and grains. RDA for Folate is 400mcg/day, but some Naturopaths recommend 800mcg/day.

Biotin is part of the B-Family, discovered in 1942. It supports gluconeogenesis (the synthesis of glucose) and is important in carb and fat metabolism. Small amounts of Biotin are produced by gut bacteria. Biotin promotes healthy hair, skin, and nails. It is found in yeast, liver, eggs, nuts, fish, chicken, and royal jelly. RDA is 25-30mcg/day, but some Naturopaths recommend 300-500mcg/day.

B Vitamins are not typically taken alone. They work in concert with each other, so most B Vitamins are sold together.

Vitamin C (Water Soluble)

Vitamin C – Ascorbic Acid – was discovered in 1928 as a cure for scurvy. A-scorbic means without scurvy. Vitamin C is a great antioxidant. It is useful in combating cardiovascular disease. It holds the integrity of the skin, mucous membranes, and collagen. It is an immune booster and increases white blood cells. It blocks the formation of carcinogens in the blood. Vitamin C acts as a chelator to remove mercury and lead from your system. It turns iron from a less-absorbable form to a more absorbable, less reactive form. Vitamin C also acts as a Co-Enzyme in the synthesis of collagen, for certain neurotransmitters, and for liver detoxification. Things that interfere with Vitamin C include smoking, birth control pills, tetracycline, surgical procedures, and exposure to toxins. Vitamin C can be used to stop infectious diseases and help heal wounds. Vitamin C is excellent for a detox program as it aids the liver.

Vitamin D (Fat Soluble)

Vitamin D was originally discovered in 1922 as a way to cure rickets. There are different forms of Vitamin D including D2 (from plant sources) and D3 (from animal sources and cholesterol from the skin). You have Vitamin D receptors in your brain, intestines, bones, pancreas, and immune cells. The primary function of Vitamin D is calcium and phosphorus metabolism. Calcium affects your heart and muscle contraction. Your teeth and your bones rely on Vitamin D for support. Sources of Vitamin D include sunshine, cod liver oil, chicken liver, butter, egg yolks, and sardines. Although the RDA for

Vitamin D is 400 IU, some Naturopaths suggest 600 IU would be better. Vitamin D has been getting popular with medical doctors, as well. Recently, I've seen allopathic doctors prescribing as much as 2,000-4,000 IU of Vitamin D.

Vitamin E (Fat Soluble)

Vitamin E was discovered in 1924 and functions primarily as a fat-soluble anti-oxidant. That means it needs fat to be effective. As an anti-oxidant, it kills free-radicals.   It works in fatty regions of the body such as adipose tissue and cell membranes (and cell membrane health is key in overall health.) Vitamin E also has an anti-clotting function that helps to thin the blood. It may be good for fighting heart disease and lower cholesterol. The natural form of Vitamin E is called "D-alpha" tocopherol. The synthetic form, "DL" is unnatural and only about half as potent. The synthetic forms are epsilon, eta, zeta, or mixed. Of course, I always recommend the natural version. Check your labels! Vitamin E is actually not a single chemical. It has eight components:

Tocopherols	Tocotrienols
Alpha	Alpha
Beta	Beta
Gamma	Gamma
Delta	Delta

Tocotrienols were discovered in 1964 but their benefits weren't fully known until the 1980's. Recently, studies have been done that utilize tocotrienols for pancreatic, breast, prostate, liver, and skin cancers.

Vitamin E can be depleted by stress, pollution, toxins, and processed foods. If you lack Vitamin E, you may get cold fingers and toes, swelling of the face, ankles, and legs, muscle cramps, and poor skin.

Sources of Vitamin E include: Wheat germ oil, nuts & seeds, unrefined vegetable oil. The richest source of tocotrienols is found in virgin crude palm oil. The RDA for Vitamin E is 400 IU or 15mg

(I've seen both).   Tocotrienols, by themselves, have been supplemented from 40-360mg per day.

Vitamin F

Vitamin F is an outdated term for the essential fatty acids Omega-3 and Omega-6, which we discussed earlier. I'm not sure if anyone is still using the term Vitamin F.

Vitamin K (Fat Soluble)

Vitamin K was discovered in 1935 and it acts as a clotting agent on proteins in the body. It is one of the fat-soluble vitamins. It is measured in micrograms (not milligrams or IU). It helps with the recovery of wounds and injuries, and it is helpful for your bones. You need healthy bacteria in your gut in order to synthesize Vitamin K. People who need Vitamin K are those who have issues such as colitis, diarrhea, and even cancer. If you don't have enough Vitamin K, you may bruise easily and bleed easily.

The RDA for Vitamin K is 45-80mcg, but some Naturopaths recommend as much as 500mcg for prevention and as much as 5-10mg for people with osteoporosis (of course, you should consult with your doctor.) Vitamin K can be found in green vegetables, broccoli, and in your gut bacteria. If you take antibiotics, it will kill your gut flora which will reduce the Vitamin K in your body.

Hopefully, by now you can see how incredibly important vitamins are for you and why I recommend them.

Minerals

Minerals are important, as well.

I don't want to go over every mineral, but I will go through some of the more important ones.

There are some essential minerals including: iron, zinc, copper, iodine, manganese, chromium, molybdenum, selenium, and some non-essential and possibly toxic minerals including: gold, silver, aluminum, mercury, cadmium, lead, and beryllium.

Macro Minerals include: calcium, phosphorus, magnesium, sodium, potassium, chloride, sulfur, and silicon.

Micro Minerals (trace minerals) include all of the essential and non-essential minerals listed above.

It is very important not only to look at the minerals themselves, but also the ratio between certain minerals. There are minerals that work together and interact together, and sometimes the ratios can be more important than the amount of each individual mineral.

Calcium

Calcium is the most abundant mineral in your body. Most of your calcium (99%) resides in your bones and teeth, and only about 1% is in your blood, but your calcium is very important and has many functions. That one percent regulates muscle contraction, cell permeability, release of neurotransmitters, and clotting. Calcium is regulated by hormones and is one of the materials used to manufacture cortisone, estrogen, and androgen. Calcium affects your bones, nervous system, muscles, circulatory system, digestive system, and immune system. Parathyroid Hormone increases absorption and calcitonin decreases absorption. Organic calcium is seen as calcium citrate, ascorbate, and aspartate. Inorganic calcium is seen as calcium carbonate. If you are acidic, it will cause depletion of calcium. Hydrochloric acid in the stomach is needed for calcium absorption. Older people and people taking acid inhibitors don't have as much HCl and therefore have less ability to absorb calcium. Vitamin D and magnesium are also needed for calcium absorption, which is why you'll often see them sold together. Until recently, the ratio of magnesium to calcium was set as 1:2. Things are beginning to change, so keep your eye on new studies. Sometimes, calcium is used as therapy for osteoporosis, blood pressure, muscle cramps, insomnia, and anxiety. Moderate exercise also helps absorb calcium and helps strengthen bone. Calcium can be found in broccoli, sea vegetables, sesame seeds, yogurt, and Kefir. (Milk also has calcium, but I'm not a big fan of milk for a number of reasons.) RDA is 750 mg, although some Naturopaths recommend 1000-1300mg/day.

Magnesium

Magnesium works in conjunction with Calcium. It keeps calcium dissolved in the blood. Magnesium in its organic form is seen as magnesium citrate, aspartate, and glycenate. The inorganic form can be seen as magnesium oxide and chloride. Magnesium can be found in nuts, seeds, pumpkin seeds, legumes, green veggies, Brewer's yeast, kelp, and whole grains. Magnesium is the building block of bones. Sixty percent of magnesium goes into bone. It is also a co-factor for over 300 enzymes in the body. The processing of food removes magnesium. Too much magnesium leads to diarrhea, which is why it is used in many constipation and colon cleanse products. If you drink a lot of coffee, take diuretics, or sweat a lot, you could be losing magnesium. Magnesium is sometimes used as therapy for constipation, cramping, esophageal spasms, asthma, and heart disease. It is anti-thrombic (helps your heart) and anti-clotting. It can lower blood pressure by relaxing smooth muscle. It can also raise your good HDL cholesterol. Your heart contains eighteen times more magnesium than your blood. A lack of magnesium could lead to arrhythmia. RDA for magnesium is 320-420mg/day, but some Naturopaths recommend 750mg/day.

Sodium

Sodium is one of the main electrolytes in the body. It is found in the watery parts of the body. It regulates the fluid balance in your body. Sodium chloride (salt) causes water retention and increases blood pressure. Sodium and potassium work together to regulate nerve cell conduction. A good sodium to potassium ratio might be 3:1 but with the usual Standard American Diet, we probably aren't even close. Many people tend to think that sodium is the same as salt (sodium chloride), but that is untrue. Your body needs sodium.

49

Sodium helps with nerve impulses, muscle contraction, and nutrient metabolism. Celery is a great source of natural, organic sodium. Of course, too much salt (NaCl) is not good for you and could lead to hypertension, water retention, edema, weak muscles, fatigue, and problems with your liver and pancreas.

Potassium

Potassium works in conjunction with Sodium as an electrolyte. Together, they help carry nutrients into cells while at the same time removing waste products. Potassium helps the thyroid gland and helps regulate the acidity in the blood and bodily fluids. If your body is too acidic, it will cause your kidneys to excrete potassium and water, which will cause you to become dehydrated. Blood pressure drugs that act as diuretics cause the body to lose potassium. Any type of diuretic such as coffee, tea, soda, and alcohol will deplete your potassium. Lack of potassium can cause blood sugar disorders and muscle cramps. Your potassium to sodium ratio should be 1:3. You can get your potassium from green leafy vegetables.

Sodium/Potassium Ratio

You can't talk about sodium or potassium without discussing the importance of the ratio between the two. They need each other to work effectively. A good sodium to potassium ratio is 3:1. If the ratio is above 10 or less than 1.5, it could lead to serious issues with your liver, kidneys, and immune system. Sodium is more associated with the adrenals, whereas potassium is associated with the thyroid. Studies have shown that the sodium/potassium ratio may be more important than the amount of sodium or potassium alone. That's pretty huge. How do you get the best sodium/potassium ratio? It shouldn't surprise you when I tell you that you should eat less packaged, processed food, and eat more fresh whole foods. There is also a link between a high sodium/potassium ratio with a zinc and/or magnesium deficiency. Zinc tends to lower sodium levels while raising potassium. Similarly, magnesium lowers sodium levels.

Conversely, copper, mercury, and cadmium toxicity will raise sodium levels and reduce potassium levels.

Phosphorus

Normally, we consume too much phosphorus due to the additives in sodas. It is the second most abundant mineral in the body. Eighty percent of phosphorus is held in the bones and teeth. Phosphorus is used not only for bones and teeth but also nerves, muscles, and energy metabolism. It is necessary for the formation of bile and lipoproteins (fat carriers) that keep fat from sticking to your arterial walls, thus avoiding atherosclerosis. We don't normally lack Phosphorus. Too much Phosphorus will leach calcium from your bones. It can also lead to kidney stones. It is found in meat, fish, nuts, eggs, legumes, and grains. Phosphorus and sulfur form acid in the body. Phosphorus actually glows in the dark when exposed to air!

Zinc

The inorganic form of zinc is in the form of zinc sulfate, oxide, and chloride. The organic form of zinc is in the form of zinc aspartate or piccolinate. Zinc works with copper and should be balanced in an 8:1 ratio of zinc to copper. It is a co-factor for over seventy enzymes in the body. Zinc is needed for HCl production in the stomach which activates pepsin. Zinc is needed to release Vitamin A from the liver and for proper immune function. It is also necessary for insulin function, proper growth of skin cells, regulation of prostate cells, and proper manufacture of RNA and DNA. Zinc plays a role in protein production, carbon dioxide transport, circulatory system, fat metabolism, bones, joints, eyes, and the production of sex hormones. Zinc is often used to fight colds and flu (Ie. Zinc lozenges). Zinc can be found in oysters, meat, fish, poultry, pumpkin seeds, legumes, whole grains, eggs, and Swiss chard. RDA is 12-15mg/day, but some Naturopaths recommend 20-25mg/day.

Copper

Copper functions as a co-factor for the anti-oxidant SOD, helps lower cholesterol, affects blood vessel strength, and helps with connective tissue synthesis (similar to Vitamin C). A copper deficiency could lead to osteoporosis, cardiovascular disease, stroke, and muscle weakness. Too much copper can be toxic. We may get too much copper from copper pipes and pots and pans. Too much copper could trigger migraines.

Chromium

Chromium is often used in weight-loss programs, because of its function of metabolizing carbs. It enhances the activity of insulin and helps get glucose into the cells. Chromium is found in Glucose Tolerance Factor (GTF) which is needed by insulin to allow cells to absorb glucose. It is a factor in the immune system, the liver, and the adrenal glands. The inorganic form is chromium chloride. The organic form is chromium piccolinate, which is better absorbed. Diets high in sugar use up more chromium. Chromium has been used for cardiovascular disease, hypo and hyper glycemia, and also used to increase lean muscle mass. Chromium is found in many foods including mushrooms, green leafy vegetables, root vegetables, chicken, seafood, whole wheat, brewer's yeast, black pepper, and fresh fruit and fruit juice. RDA for Chromium is 50mcg.

Selenium

Selenium was once thought to be toxic, but now it's known as a powerful antioxidant that acts as a free-radical scavenger. This should make you realize that what is set in stone today may change tomorrow. Selenium helps protect your heart, red blood cells, eyes, and prostate. It is needed in protein synthesis. The inorganic form is sodium selenite and sodium selenate. The organic form is selenomethionine and selenocysteine. Selenium is part of glutathioneperoxidase. It governs your metabolic process by converting T4 (Thyroxin) to T3. A deficiency can lead to heart disease and cancer. It is also often used in various Detox programs.

Selenium can be found in fish, organ meats, oats, Brazil nuts, grains, asparagus, onions, tomatoes, garlic, and veggies. RDA is 50-70mcg/day, but Naturopaths often recommend up to 200mcg/day.

Iron

Iron used to be considered essential, but now can be potentially toxic. Another example of how things change as we get more information. The inorganic form of iron is iron sulfate. The organic form is iron citrate or iron glycanate. Iron can be found in liver, oysters, tofu, amaranth, lentils, Swiss chard, and sea vegetables. Iron acts as a co-factor for many enzymes. Most people these days do not have a deficiency in iron unless you have heavy blood loss, bleeding ulcer, or heavy menstrual cycle. RDA is 10-15mg/day.

Iodine

Iodine is key in keeping your thyroid gland healthy, and your thyroid gland affects your metabolism. Your metabolism is important in weight loss. The inorganic form of iodine is potassium iodide. Organic iodine can be found in sea vegetables, seafood, and iodine is typically added to salt. Most people in the U.S. are not overly deficient in iodine, but a deficiency can lead to goiter due to a thyroid problem. If you have hypothyroidism or goiter, you may want to consider taking iodine. RDA is 150mcg.

Manganese

Manganese is essential in the formation of connective tissue and acts as a co-factor for the anti-oxidant SOD. Manganese is an ingredient in bile which is needed for fat metabolism. It also is necessary for protein metabolism. It works with Vitamin K in blood clotting and it works with zinc to raise low blood pressure. Manganese works with your skeletal system and your immune system as well as helping your brain and nerves. The inorganic form is manganese chloride. The organic form is manganese citrate. Manganese has been used for people with osteoporosis, arthritis, atherosclerosis, diabetes, and possibly epilepsy. Manganese can be found in whole grains, pecans, Brazil nuts, pumpkin seeds, peanuts, bananas, blueberries, and blackberries.

Chapter 6 – Enzymes

There are hundreds of enzymes in your body. Why are they so important? If fats and proteins are the raw materials and carbs are the energy source in our bodies, enzymes are the workers that make everything happen. Without enzymes, there would be no chemical reactions. Our bodies manufacture approximately 24 digestive enzymes. Earlier, I mentioned that raw foods have enzymes which help in the digestive process. Enzymes in food have the ability to "self-digest" the food which contains it. Enzymes are the catalysts that allow all chemical reactions in the body to take place. Vitamins, minerals, carbs, fats, and proteins are all activated by enzymes. This circles back around to our discussion about the efficacy of vitamins. One of the reasons your vitamins may not be working is due to a lack of enzymes.

Food enzymes share the responsibility of digestion with enzymes produced in the body. Keep in mind that cooking/heating destroys enzymes, and the Standard American Diet of processed foods has very little, if any, enzymes. If you're not eating raw foods with enzymes, it places all the burden of digestion on your body alone. The organs in your body that produce enzymes are simply not capable of producing enough enzymes. A deficiency in enzymes leads to chronic health issues. According to Dr. Howard F. Loomis,

"If food enzymes do some of the work, the body is not burdened with eliminating an accumulation of food it cannot assimilate. Food allergies, gas and bloating, heartburn, constipation, or diarrhea are only minor problems that can result. Studies are gradually revealing that the resulting metabolic problems may be the direct cause of many chronic degenerative diseases." (Enzymes, The Key to Health)

The thought is that if we don't eat enough enzymes; the body has to steal enzymes from other parts of the body which causes a competition among the other organs in your body, and this may lead to obesity and degenerative diseases.

All living things contain enzymes including plants and animals. Some enzymes work in an acidic environment, while other enzymes only work in an alkaline environment. Enzyme supplements made from animal enzymes come from the pancreas of beef and pork. On the label, you'll see this as Pancreatin. Animal enzymes only work in an alkaline environment, therefore only work in the intestines, not in the stomach. Food enzymes work in the stomach which actually means the enzymes are able to "pre-digest" food in your stomach. Food enzymes are able to digest as much as 60% of starch, 30% of protein, and 10% of fat, before the food reaches your intestines. (Enzymes, The Key to Health, p. 68)

Where do enzymes work? You have enzymes in your mouth. Your salivary glands secrete enzymes. If you are eating raw foods, enzymes are released from the food in the mouth, as well. Once the food enters your stomach, the food enzymes and salivary enzymes continue to work. Studies have shown that 45% of carbs can be digested in the stomach within 15 minutes with only salivary amylase. (Enzymes, The Key to Health, p. 87)

This next statement may shock you. **Hydrochloric acid in the stomach does not digest food!** The acid in your stomach only creates the environment for digestion to take place. Think about that for a minute. When you have acid stomach, what do you take or what does the doctor prescribe? Acid inhibitors. Pills or drinks to shut down acid production. When you shut down acid production, the enzymes don't digest the food, and the food moves through into your intestines undigested. Undigested food sits in your gut and begins to putrefy. Vitamins and minerals are not absorbed. All this can lead to constipation, bloating, gas, and eventually will become diseases such as Crohn's, diverticulitis, colitis, and cancer. By the way, I have read from multiple sources that enzymes have the ability to "digest" cancer cells by eating away the protein coating surrounding cancer cells, but we'll have to leave that discussion for another book.

Dr. Richard Anderson classifies enzymes this way:

Enzymes are categorized by their function (s):

- **Metabolic enzymes** *catalyze and regulate every biochemical reaction that occurs in your body and are essential to cellular function and health.*

- **Digestive enzymes** *are secreted along the digestive tract, break down food into nutrients and waste, and allow the nutrients found in foods to be absorbed into the bloodstream. The pancreas produces most digestive enzymes, but the liver, gallbladder, small intestines, stomach and colon also play critical roles in the production of these enzymes. Examples of digestive enzymes: lipase, protease, amylase, ptyalin, pepsin and trypsin.*

- **Food enzymes** *enter the body through the consumption of raw foods or enzyme supplements. Cooking and processing destroys most enzymes in food.*

- **Plant Based enzymes** *are synthetically grown, help break down fat, protein and carbohydrates and function within a broad pH range. Plant enzymes, commonly Bromelin (pineapple) and Papain (papaya) play an important role in more complete digestion of all foods. They are activated at a temperature higher than normal body temperature, also making them a good anti-inflammatory.*

- **Proteolytic enzymes** *are enzymes that digest proteins, including Trypsin, Chymotrypsin, Pancreatin, Bromelin and Papain. Some are produced by the pancreas and others are supplemental from animals or plants. The primary use of proteolytic enzymes in supplements is as digestive aid. They are also used in drugs as anti-inflammatory agents and pain relievers.*

Dr. Anderson also says the following about enzymes and non-raw foods:

Food should not deplete or rob the body of its needed essence or harm it in any way. Dead or dying foods take an enormous toll on the body. Consider these facts about cooked, frozen, canned, and processed foods:

- *They have been depleted of many vitamins*
- *They create toxins*
- *They drain the life force from the body*
- *They harm the constructive bacteria in the intestines*
- *They produce harmful bacteria in the intestines*
- *They poison the bloodstream, thereby feeding disease*
- *They clog the body's lymph system*
- *They drain the body's enzyme reserve*
- *They overwork and clog the elimination systems*
- *They strain the glandular system, especially the endocrine glands*
- *They overwork the digestive system*
- *They cause stress, congestion and mucus*
- *They produce the ideal environment for parasites*
- *They lower our consciousness, our spiritual vibration.*

*(*www.ariseandshine.com*)*

With that knowledge, you may want to consider eating more raw fruits and vegetables rather than cooked and processed foods.

It is also very important to remember that in order for enzymes to work, they need to be in the right pH environment. Different enzymes work in different pH environments. Enzymes in the stomach only work in an acidic environment. Enzymes in the intestines only work in alkaline environment.

Chapter 7 - Probiotics

There was an article out recently in which Dr. Oz was asked what his best approach for dieting was. His number one best weight loss approach is using probiotics. Yes, something that Naturopaths have been talking about for years is just now beginning to go mainstream. That's a positive sign that medicine is moving in the right direction. Of course, there are good bacteria and bad bacteria. Dr. Oz calls them fat bacteria and skinny bacteria. I would guess that most people have an overabundance of bad bacteria and not enough good bacteria. Bad bacteria grows when we eat processed foods, (bad) carbs, sugar, and (bad) fats. Also, when you take antibiotics, that will kill off the bad bacteria, but it will also kill off your good bacteria. Having too much bad bacteria and not enough good bacteria will lead to weight gain, poor digestion, bloating, intestinal issues, and yeast infections. I would highly suggest using prebiotics and probiotics to rebuild the good bacteria in your gut. This will help tremendously not only with your weight loss but also with other intestinal issues.

There are certain foods that are good for your intestinal flora. Fermented foods help. Studies have shown that regular consumption of fermented foods can not only correct digestive problems, but also have positive effects on heart disease, arthritis, obesity, gum disease, mood and more. (http://www.naturalnews.com)

Probiotics have the following benefits:

- Supports your immune system
- Supports digestion
- Promotes bowel regularity
- Assists nutrient absorption and assimilation
- Relieves gas
- Supports a healthy pH level in your gut
- Fights yeast infections
- Relieves bloating and constipation
- Reduces cholesterol in the blood
- Reduces unhealthy bacteria and yeast in the intestines

- Reduces high blood pressure
- Assists in elimination ailments such as constipation, colitis, irritable bowel syndrome, and acne
- Produces natural anti-bacterial agents (antibiotics)
- Can help calcium assimilation
- Can help detoxify chemicals added to foods

According to Dr. Richard Anderson, the most dangerous enemies of your friendly bacteria are:

- Drugs – especially antibiotics, since one dose can eliminate all friendly bacteria
- Alcohol – destroys friendly bacteria and enzymes, not to mention actual cells
- Pasteurized dairy products are gourmet meals for pathogens which destroy the good bacteria
- Cooked meat – it feeds the bacillus E. coli and other pathogens
- Bread – especially white flour or any wheat products that were baked in an oven (wheat is only good in its raw, sprouted state)
- White sugar – chocolate, cakes, pies, cookies, pop, catsup, etc.
- Fried foods – e.g. potato chips, French fries, and anything fried in oil
- Acid-forming foods, when overused
- Processed foods, such as pasta; all the food in packages

(Cleanse and Purify Thyself, Dr. Richard Anderson, p 110)

Chapter 8 - Digestion – Putting it all together

Your digestion begins the minute you jam that food into your mouth. (Actually, digestion begins in your brain the minute you see or smell the food in front of you.) The first thing you do is start chewing. Chewing breaks the food down into smaller pieces, which makes it easier to digest. By chewing your food, it increases the amount of surface space available for enzymes to begin their process. As a side note, if you're one of those people who gets gas when eating vegetables, it may be because you're not chewing your veggies enough. Vegetables are covered in cellulose. Cooking breaks down the cellulose, but if you're eating raw veggies, then you basically have to chew off the cellulose. Chewing also slows down the entire eating process. Many people eat too fast. Are you one of those people? Eating slowly is very important to good digestion. The saliva in your mouth does a couple of things. It moistens the food particles in your mouth and saliva also produces digestive enzymes including amylase which digests carbs, protease which digests protein, and lipase which digests fat. At the same time, the enzymes in food also begin working on digesting the food.

Stomach

Once you swallow the food, it goes down your throat (pharynx and esophagus) into your stomach. It takes about 45 minutes for your stomach to begin producing hydrochloric acid. If you remember, the hydrochloric acid allows the enzymes in your stomach to continue the digestion process. Gastric acid also kills bacteria that enters with the food. If you are taking antacids, you are probably doing more harm than good. If you cancel out the acid, the enzymes won't be able to digest the food, and the food will continue into your intestines undigested, which could lead to a variety of health issues. Turning off your gastric acids also allow bacteria to enter into your gut. If you want to lose weight, you need to make sure your body is producing hydrochloric acid and digesting properly. On a side note, you need enough protein in your system to produce HCl, and you need enough organic sodium to protect your stomach lining from the HCl.

Small Intestine

As the food passes from the stomach into the duodenum, the first part of the small intestines, the pancreas produces more enzymes to help digest carbs, protein, and fats. The more your food is pre-digested before entering the intestines, the less work the pancreas has to do. As mentioned earlier, stomach enzymes work in an acidic environment, but enzymes in the duodenum need an alkaline environment. The mucosal tissue of the small intestines is alkaline with a pH of about 8.5. The pancreas also helps in that area by producing bicarbonate. Eighty-five percent of all nutrients are absorbed through your small intestine. It is in the small intestine where your vitamins, minerals, and water are absorbed. Most absorption and digestion should be complete by the middle of the small intestine.

Liver and Gall Bladder

Your liver and gallbladder also play an important role in digestion. Your liver is in charge of handling the glucose in your system. If you remember, too much glucose not only causes an insulin response, but glucose gets transformed into fat. Fat molecules are difficult to digest. Bile is able to emulsify fat molecules which then allows the enzymes to break it down. If you don't have bile production, you won't be able to digest fat efficiently, and it will also lead to gas. Bile is produced by the liver and stored in the gallbladder. Bile contains both cholesterol and sodium. Oftentimes, when you don't have enough stomach acid (due to lack of sodium and/or protein), you will have gallbladder issues. Also, if you lose weight too quickly, your gall bladder could accumulate and store bile which could turn to gall stones. So it is important to eat right and take supplements to avoid that. (As you can see, your body is a pretty complex piece of machinery where a number of different things from different systems are all working together.) The liver ultimately metabolizes the fats, carbs, and protein molecules.

Large Intestine

Believe it or not, did you know that 90% of all cells in the human body are bacteria that live in the large intestine! What does that mean for you? If you ask a Naturopath, they will most likely tell you that all disease starts in the gut. That's a pretty powerful statement. According to Dr. Howard Loomis, *"...maintenance of a normal bacterial flora is imperative for health. Auto-intoxication (lack of adequate intestinal flora) is the underlying cause of an exceptionally large group of symptom complexes."* The microflora in your gut affects nutrition, infection, metabolism, and toxicity. As with everything else we've talked about, there is both good bacteria and bad bacteria.

Insulin

We've spoken earlier about the insulin response. Insulin is a hormone that was discovered in 1921. It plays a key role in sugar metabolism. Insulin is what takes the sugar in your blood and allows it to enter into your cells for storage for later use. When you eat a high carb meal, the flood of sugar into your system causes the pancreas to release insulin which takes the sugar out of your blood and puts it into your cells which brings your blood sugar levels back down. If your blood sugar drops too much, you become hypoglycemic. If you're working out at the gym, and you start to feel light-headed, it may be that your blood sugar is too low. An excess of sugar stored in your cells becomes fat. If your insulin levels remain high, it will be difficult to lose weight, because insulin inhibits the breakdown of fat. In short, obesity is probably the most common result of insulin resistance. Therefore, it is important to eat a healthy meal that does not cause an insulin response. Additionally, once you have an insulin response, it triggers your brain to create serotonin which is what makes you feel tired after a large carb diet.

In Conclusion

If you want to lose weight and enjoy all the benefits that come along with weight loss including increased energy, better mood, better skin, reduced aches and pains, and reduced risk of disease; the key is in having a good digestive system and proper assimilation. Why? Because your gut is where you absorb nutrients and get rid of waste. You know the old saying, "you are what you eat," but in reality, it should be, "you are what you absorb." If your intestines are all blocked up, not only will you gain weight, but you will not be able to absorb nutrients, you'll have too much bad bacteria in your system, and you won't be getting rid of the junk in your system. A healthy system will be able to absorb nutrients and get rid of waste. An unhealthy system will not absorb nutrients and will not excrete waste.

Chapter 9 - Fasting and Detox for Weight Loss

People often have a misconception of fasting, cleansing, and detoxification. Fasting is not meant to be a weight loss program. If you fast, you will lose weight. If you fast you will detox. But if you return to your normal, standard American diet and lifestyle after your fast, you will gain all the weight back. Fasting is meant to be therapeutic for healing. According to Dr. Dharma Singh Khalsa, M.D. the benefits from fasting include:

- During a fast the body rids itself of damaged, diseased, aged, and dead cells

- The rate of new healthy cell growth is increased

- The capacity of the lungs, liver, kidneys, and skin is greatly increased, and masses of wastes and toxins are eliminated

- Fasting allows digestive, assimilative, and protective organs to rest

- Fasting exerts normalizing, stabilizing, and rejuvenating effects on vital physiological and mental functions

- Fasting normalizes your relationship with food

    (Food as Medicine, Dharma Singh Khalsa, M.D. p 73)

Fasting has been used for thousands of years around the globe by such people as Socrates, Plato, Pythagoras, and Hippocrates. There have been numerous books written on the beneficial effects of fasting, and I suggest you read some of them. In today's world, there are a lot of naysayers who say that fasting is bad for multiple reasons. I'm in the camp that thinks fasting is an amazing way to heal your body. According to Dr. Joel Fuhrman, M.D.:

"Therapeutic fasting accelerates the healing process and allows the body to recover from serious disease in a dramatically short period of time. In my practice I have seen fasting eliminate lupus and arthritis, remove chronic skin conditions such as psoriasis and

eczema, heal the digestive tract in patients with ulcerative colitis and Crohn's disease, and quickly eliminate cardiovascular diseases such as high blood pressure and angina. "

Dr. William Esser stated, *"In a fast we can observe the body gleefully going about getting rid of the toxins and wastes accumulated for years with the greatest capability and intelligence, all on its own."*

The reason fasting works is because it allows the body to detoxify. The more "bad" foods we eat, the more toxic our system becomes. Toxins can be in the form of oxidized fats, cholesterol, free radicals, etc. But food is not the only source of toxins. Amalgam fillings made with mercury can lead to mercury poisoning. Drugs, both illegal and pharmaceutical, can be toxic to your system. If you don't believe me, read the small print on the drugs the doctor prescribes for you. Pharmaceuticals are inherently toxic to your liver. Detoxing the body allows you to clear out the excess mucus, congestion, fat, and other toxins, which can reduce inflammation and balance your pH. Poor digestion and elimination hinders your body's effort to detoxify. In a healthy body, detoxification is a natural process. Your body will detoxify through the lungs, skin, kidneys, lymph system, and bowels. Your liver is the chief detoxifier in your body.

Paul C. Bragg (famous for Bragg's Apple Cider Vinegar) put it this way,

"Fasting works by self-digestion. During a fast your body intuitively will decompose and burn only the substances and tissues that are damaged, diseased or unneeded, such as abscesses, tumors, excess fat deposits, excess water and congestive wastes. Even a short fast (1-3 days) will accelerate eliminations from your liver, kidneys, lungs, bloodstream and skin. Sometimes you will experience dramatic changes (cleansing and healing crisis) as accumulated wastes are expelled. With your first fasts you may temporarily have cleansing headaches, fatigue, body odor, bad breath, coated tongue, mouth sores and even diarrhea as your body is cleaning house. Please be patient with your body."

How do you know if you are toxic and need to detox? Here is a list of symptoms of toxicity:

Headaches	*Backaches*	*Runny Nose*	*Fatigue*
Joint Pain	*Itchy Nose*	*Nervousness*	*Anxiety*
Skin Rash	*Cough*	*Frequent Colds*	*Sleepiness*
Hives	*Wheezing*	*Irritated Eyes*	*Insomnia*
Nausea	*Sore Throat*	*Immune Weakness*	*Dizziness*
Indigestion	*Stiff Neck*	*Allergies*	*Mood Changes*
Anorexia	*Angina*	*Sinus Congestion*	*Fever*
Bad Breath	*Depression*	*Constipation*	*Poor Circulation*

(Staying Healthy with Nutrition, Elson M. Haas, p.908)

Are there different types of fasting? Technically, fasting means not eating anything and only consuming water. Your body is either consuming or expelling, with absorption going on in between. A fast will allow your body to give 100% effort to expelling. There are some people who think fasting is unsafe. Maybe in today's world, with the sad state of health many people are in, maybe that is true. But generally speaking, your body should be able to do a fast.

If you don't want to do a 100% water fast, there are a myriad of different things you can do that are still considered a fast and detox. You can add certain things to your fast that may help the detox process while not using your digestive system too much. For example, you can take certain herbs that will help cleanse and detox the liver, gallbladder, and kidneys. You can take flax seeds or chia seeds (whole or ground) to help clear out the colon. You can take bentonite clay which draws toxins out of the colon. These are a few things you can do. You can also do a juice fast, which we will cover in the next section. If you're going to do a water fast, you can do a pre-fast for three days where you may want to do a juice fast or eat just fruits and vegetables prior to the water fast. It will make your fast a little easier.

How long should you fast? That's entirely up to you. I would say a three-day fast is a good start. Anything less than that will probably not be enough time. A friend of mine fasted for thirty days, and he loved it. The first two to three days of a fast will be the most difficult. During that time, you will be going through withdrawals from mostly sugar and caffeine. You may get headaches, feel tired and achy, be restless, and you'll probably be cranky. But I always tell people it's like going through a tunnel. Once you get to the other side, you'll have more energy, you'll have less aches and pains, you'll be able to think more clearly, and you'll probably weigh about 10lbs less. From that point, you have to begin eating healthy and make sure you don't fall back into your old eating habits.

Here is one thing to consider, also. There is a difference between fasting and doing some kind of fad diet. When you diet, you are always hungry – especially if you're doing a low fat or low carb diet. But when you fast, after about the third day, you no longer have food cravings! As far as weight loss goes, people have lost from seven to twenty pounds within the first seven to ten days of fasting. Of course, everyone is different, but I personally lost nine pounds doing a three-day juice fast.

Lastly, I just want to clarify some terms. I use "cleanse" and "detox" interchangeably. Some people separate the two and define them differently. The one thing I will say is that I would suggest doing a colon "cleanse" before doing a liver "detox". The reason behind that thinking is that if you detox your liver, you will be dumping a lot of toxins into your colon for removal, and if your colon is all clogged up, you will only recirculate the toxins throughout your system. Therefore, you should always detox your colon before anything else.

Chapter 10 - Juicing

Juicing is one of my favorite things. It is an excellent way to get your vitamins, minerals, and enzymes all in one. In massive quantities. Of course, there are those people who will tell you why juicing is not good for you, but their logic doesn't hold much water. Juice fasting is a form of detoxification. Let's begin with the fruits and vegetables all at once. You wouldn't be able to get that amount of vitamins and minerals by eating those foods in a meal. Most people are hard-pressed to get in a couple of fruits and vegetables every day. For example, when I juice, I usually use a couple apples, a few carrots, a few stalks of celery, one or two beets, a handful of kale, a handful of spinach, a handful of cilantro, a whole cucumber, and a thumb size of ginger. Most people won't sit down and eat that. Another good thing about juicing is that unlike eating the whole fruit or vegetable which takes longer to digest, juicing gets into your system quickly without the need for much digestion. This gives your digestive system a break.

You can add juicing to your daily routine and substitute your coffee, sodas, or fruit drink with fresh juices. Or you can try a 3-5 day juice fast which has numerous health benefits.

The naysayers usually have a few arguments. The first argument against juicing is that you're taking the fiber out of the fruits and vegetables. This is quite true. And yes, fiber is very important to your health as it serves as the scrubbing bubbles to keep your intestines cleaned out. But we're not juicing for the fiber. We're juicing for the vitamins, minerals, and enzymes. I always recommend eating fresh raw fruits and vegetables also in order to get your fiber. The second argument is the sugar argument. If you juice so many fruits and vegetables all at once, won't that spike your blood sugar and cause an insulin response. Earlier, you read where the fructose from fruits and vegetables does NOT cause an insulin response, according to Dr. Hoffer. If you want to play it safe, I suggest monitoring your blood sugar with a glucose monitor when you're juicing, and see how it affects your own blood sugar levels, and see how you feel.

I just read a report recently that said drinking fruit juice was no better than drinking sodas because of the sugar content in juice. Did they differentiate between fresh fruit juice and processed fruit juice you buy in cans and bottles? No, of course not. I agree that processed juices have a super-high sugar content. But I'm not advocating drinking massive amounts of processed juices. When we're talking about drinking juice, I mean fresh juice that you make in your home from the fruit itself. When you read reports like that, always delve into what they're saying, so you don't get the wrong information.

When you are doing a juice fast, you will lose weight while at the same time loading up your body with an abundance of vitamins, minerals and enzymes. The third argument against juicing is that you're only losing water weight, and you'll gain it all back when you start eating again. I've had heated conversations with my friends about this. When I juiced for three days, I lost nine pounds. A week after I started eating again, I had gained three pounds back. But I have to say, I wasn't eating totally healthy. My wife brought home a box of apple turnovers, which I had to eat, of course.

If I had returned to a healthy diet, I probably would not have gained any more weight. More importantly, fruits and vegetables are made up of primarily water. I'll attach a list in the appendix section for you to look at. If fruits and vegetables are mostly water mixed with vitamins, minerals, enzymes, and fiber, if we take out the fiber and drink the juice, we're basically drinking fresh vitamin water. Here is a good example. The water content of carrot juice is almost identical to the water content in fresh milk. The difference is that milk forms mucus in your body and has a large amount of casein. Casein is a milk by-product that is used in making glue. Carrot juice, on the other hand has a plethora of healthy benefits and is used in many health drinks.

Some people say that fresh juice is just concentrated food, but this is not the case. An example of concentrated food would be dried fruit, where the water has been removed, and what is left over is the concentrated food. Juices are just the opposite. They are highly un-concentrated. They are one of the least concentrated but most nourishing.

Let me list out a few vegetables and why they are good for you:

Carrot Juice – One of my favorite juices! Carrot juice is one of the best sources of beta-carotene which converts to vitamin A and also has vitamins B,C,D,E, and K. It is good for both appetite and digestion. According to Dr. Walker, raw carrot juice is a natural solvent for ulcerous and cancerous conditions. It helps prevent infections and protects the nervous system. It is helpful in cleansing the liver. Carrot juice contains sodium, potassium, calcium, magnesium, and iron. The lutein and zeaxanthin found in carrots are very helpful for the eyes. Carrots help the mucous membranes in your respiratory tract. I read that the carrot juice molecule is very similar to that of the blood molecule. That's pretty interesting. Carrot juice is full of anti-oxidants and is used in so many different juice formulas.

Celery - Raw celery contains more than four times as much organic sodium as calcium. Keep in mind that organic sodium is not salt (sodium chloride). Sodium is very important to the body. This is good for people who consume large amounts of carbohydrates. Sodium helps eliminate carbon dioxide from the system. Sodium is one of the main ingredients in bile which is needed for digestion of fats. Sodium also protects the stomach from HCl. Celery is also high in magnesium and iron which is food for blood cells. Celery and carrot juice are an excellent combo.

Cucumber - Cucumber juice is probably one of the best natural diuretics. Because of its high silicon and sulfur content, it's also good for hair and nails. Cucumber contains potassium, sodium, calcium, phosphorus, and chlorine. Mixed with carrot juice, it can alleviate rheumatic conditions. The high potassium content helps with blood pressure as well as teeth and gum issues.

Parsley - Technically, parsley is an herb, not a vegetable. It is one of the most potent juices and should not be taken alone. It is beneficial in oxygen metabolism and helps maintain the adrenal and thyroid glands. It is very good for the genito-urinary tract which helps in conditions of the kidneys and bladder. It is also very helpful for the eyes and optic nerve system. Combined with carrot, beet, and cucumber, it's also good for menstrual cramps.

Spinach - Spinach is one of the best vegetables for the entire digestive tract including the stomach, duodenum, small intestines, and large intestines. It is great for cleansing, reconstruction, and regeneration of the intestinal tract and is helpful for constipation. Spinach is high in folic acid which is good for the brain and cardiovascular system. It also contains vitamin k, quercetin (an antioxidant), manganese, magnesium, lutein, and beta-carotene. Spinach should always be eaten raw (salads or juiced.)

Beets - beets are one of the most valuable juices for helping to tone the blood. If you take too much raw beet juice (more than a wine glass), the cleansing affect may cause you to become dizzy or nauseated because of the strong cleansing effect on the liver. That's why I mix beet juice with carrot and other juices. Beet juice is a good cleanser of the liver, kidneys, gall bladder, and lymph system. Beets have beta-cyanin, which helps to fight cancer. Beets also have folic acid and potassium, which helps with metabolism and muscle function. Beets do have a relatively high sugar content and are high on the Glycemic Index, so if you're concerned about your blood sugar, you may want to monitor your blood sugar when juicing beets. I don't see an issue, though, because beet sugar is not the same as table sugar. When you're drinking beet juice, you're also getting enzymes, vitamins, and minerals which help digest the beets.

Kelp juice – Kelp is an antioxidant and anti-inflammatory that helps fight free radical damage that can cause cancer. Kelp contains iodine, folic acid, vitamin K, calcium, magnesium, and iron. The iodine in Kelp stimulates your metabolism by working on your thyroid.

Kale Juice – Kale is full of vitamins, minerals, phytonutrients, and carotenoids including vitamin C, vitamin E, beta-carotene, calcium, iron, manganese, potassium, lutein, lycopene, and zeaxanthin. Kale helps kill free radicals and protects the DNA in your genes.

You can add coconut juice to carrot, and beet juice can add flavor while still cleansing the kidneys and gall bladder. This combo contains potassium, sodium, calcium, magnesium, iron, phosphorus, sulfur, silicon, and chlorine.

Carrot, beet, cucumber juice can be used to help with gallstones, kidney stones, and gravel in the gall bladder, because it adds organic sodium and breaks down inorganic calcium deposits.

Overall, the vitamins, minerals, and live enzymes present in vegetable and fruit juicing can help with all of your health issues.

Juicing does not "treat" disease, per se, but it helps cleanse and heal your intestines, gall bladder, liver, etc. which will allow your body to heal itself, the way it was supposed to.

Now, compare that to the nutrients (or lack thereof) of the typical Standard American Diet of processed foods high in bad fats and bad carbs. I hope you're beginning to see the connection between a healthy diet and your weight and overall health.

Chapter 11 - Nutrition as Therapy

Dr. Richard O. Brennan, Chairman of the Board of Trustees, the International Academy of Preventive Medicine, says, *"Most of the food in America today will support life but it won't sustain health."* That's quite an indictment on our diet. (Putting it All Together: The New Orthomolecular Nutrition. Abram Hoffer, MD, PhD, and Morton Walker, DPM. P.15)

Dr. Hoffer also stated, *"Certain foods can prevent and cure major diseases. This has been known for hundreds of years..."*

The following is from an editorial in Nutrition Action, a newsletter of the Center for Science in the Public Interest, Washington, D.C., and reprinted in Science Magazine:

"Food faddism is promoted from birth. Sugar is a major ingredient in baby food desserts. Then come the artificially flavored and colored breakfast cereals, loaded with sugar, followed by soda pop and hot dogs. Meat marbled with fat and alcoholic beverages dominate the diets of many middle-aged people...

This diet – high in fat, sugar, cholesterol, and refined grains – is the prescription for illness; it can contribute to obesity, tooth decay, heart disease, intestinal cancer, and diabetes. And these diseases are, in fact, America's major health problems. So if any diet should be considered faddist, it is the standard one. Our far out diet – almost 20 percent refined sugar and 45 percent fat – is new to human experience and foreign to all other animal life...

It is incredible that people who eat a junk food diet constitute the norm, while individuals whose diets resemble those of our great-grandparents are labeled deviants..."

(Putting it All Together: The New Orthomolecular Nutrition. Abram Hoffer, MD, PhD, and Morton Walker, DPM. P.15)

We have gotten away from eating natural food and have become a society who eat processed foods filled with artificial preservatives and chemical additives. The key to being healthy and losing weight is to go back to eating fresh food, raw food, and food that has not been overly processed.

The Standard American Diet is associated with:

High calorie	*Low nutrient*
Low Fiber	*High Fat*
Excess Saturated Fat	*Hydrogenated Oils*
Excess Salt	*Excess Sugar*
Excess Alcohol	*Excess Milk Foods*
Excess Meats	*Excess Phosphorus*

(Staying Healthy with Nutrition, Elson M. Haas)

We want to eat exactly **opposite** of the SAD diet listed above!

Sugar

Sugar is an empty-calorie food substance. Refined sugar gives us no nutritional value. Sugar can be as addictive as heroin. Sugar is one of the leading causes of obesity, diabetes, and heart disease. And over the past few decades, we have gone from consuming 5 pounds of sugar per person per year to over 125 pounds of sugar per person per year! That's crazy! Incredibly, Americans, who make up only 5% of the world's population, consume 33% of total global sugar consumption! Sugar is only one aspect of our current American diet. Most of us are living on a junk diet. A junk diet is basically anything made with refined sugar, refined white flour, white rice, and/or alcohol. Now, refined whole wheat may also fall into this category. The amazing thing to me is that doctors have known about this for over 50 years. Way back in 1956, Surgeon-Captain T. L. Cleave, MRCP, the former director of medical research of the Institute of Naval Medicine in Great Britain said the over consumption of refined food lead to what he called the Saccharine Disease, which he defined as the Master Disease that included diabetes, coronary disease, obesity, peptic ulcer, constipation, hemorrhoids, varicose veins, E-coli, appendicitis, cholecystitis, pyelitis, diverticulitis, renal calculus, various skin conditions, and dental problems. (Putting it All Together: The New Orthomolecular Nutrition. Abram Hoffer, MD, PhD, and Morton Walker, DPM. P.22-23)

There are different types of sugar. Glucose is the energy sugar that your body and brain needs to function. Sucrose is table sugar. Eating too much sucrose can lead to high acidity, weight gain, and various physical diseases such as diabetes. Sucrose can be turned into triglycerides which gets stored as body fat. Fructose is fruit sugar and is less toxic than glucose or sucrose. According to Dr. Hoffer, **fructose does NOT stimulate the pancreas to release insulin**. That's a pretty important point for people concerned about diabetes. And since the insulin response leads to obesity, it's another reason why you should eat fruit without too much worry about sugar and weight gain. Another reason not to fear fructose from fruit is because you're not taking in just the fructose as an additive. You're also getting the enzymes and fiber.

Individual sugars can combine together to form disaccharides. They are more complex and need to be broken down by enzymes before entering the blood stream. If they are not broken down, they can sit in your gut and begin to ferment and grow bacteria. This is why enzymes and probiotics are important to sugar metabolism.

- *Sugar suppresses the immune system.*
- *Sugar elevates blood sugar.*
- *Sugar disrupts mineral balance.*
- *Sugar disrupts digestion.*
- *Sugar causes tooth decay.*
- *Sugar contributes to obesity.*
- *Sugar can cause heart disease.*
- *Sugar can cause food allergies.*
- *Sugar can cause depression.*
- *Sugar increases the risk of certain cancers.*
(www.thealternativedaily.com)

Do you go to Starbucks for a quick coffee every day? The Toronto Star examined three flavors of Frappuccino, all in the "tall" size. The Light Vanilla Frappuccino was found to contain 41 grams of sugar, which translates to 10 teaspoons. The Mocha Cookie Crumble Frappuccino contained 69 grams, or 17 teaspoons. The Caramel Ribbon Crunch Frappuccino was the worst offender, with 93 grams, or 23 teaspoons, of sugar.

(www.thealternativedaily.com)

In the end, sugar causes an insulin response which inhibits the ability of the body to burn previously stored fat. *You absolutely need to reduce your consumption of sugar.*

Whole Foods – the best diet

Whole foods are the opposite of junk food. Whole foods contain protein, fat, and carbohydrates along with vitamins and minerals. Once a food is processed, it removes much of the beneficial ingredients from the food. Processed food will never be as nutritious as whole food in its original state. Therefore, whenever possible, eat the whole food rather than the processed food. For example, eat an orange (or juice a few) rather than drinking orange juice from a carton or plastic jug. Eat brown rice instead of white rice. Eat a whole potato rather than making instant mashed potatoes or fries from a box. Fresh is better than frozen. Buy locally, if at all possible. Go down to your local farmers market. Buy things that are in season.

The best way to lose weight and be healthy is to change your diet to a healthy diet and try to avoid poor food choices and try to wean yourself off pharmaceutical drugs. You may run into some push back from your doctor, unfortunately. Doctors simply aren't sufficiently trained in nutrition during their years at medical school. One doctor said that he only received ten hours of nutritional training in four years of schooling. Also, according to an article titled, "Doctors Gamble with Rx Drugs" published in the June 1998 issue of Business & Health,

"Nearly six in ten of the 250 physicians who completed self-assessments for the American Medical Association admitted they rely solely on claims made by manufacturers' sales reps when prescribing new drugs or using new medical devices. And nearly one in seven said they don't refer to the Physicians' Desk Reference (PDR) or any other resource when they write prescriptions for other unfamiliar drugs." (Enzymes, The Key to Health, p. 138)

You also want to eat food that is organically grown. Organically grown foods have approximately 75%-350% the nutritional and mineral value of commercially grown foods. (Cancer and Natural Medicine, John Boik, p.146)

I suggest you talk to your doctor about nutrition or find a Naturopathic Doctor who understands natural health.

Soil

Your food is only as nutritious as the soil it was grown in. The food you eat gets its nutrition from the content of the soil. So if the soil is lacking nutrients, then the food is also lacking nutrients. For example, the soil in the US today is not as healthy as it was fifty or one hundred years ago. One of the reasons farmers rotate their crops is to give the land an opportunity to regenerate. Even the Bible states that you should give your land a rest every seven years. According to the Department of Agriculture, the nutritional value in food has dropped substantially since 1975:

Apples - Vitamin A is down 41%

Sweet Peppers - Vitamin C is down 31%

Watercress - Iron is down 88%

Broccoli - Calcium and Vitamin A are down 50%

Collard Greens - Vitamin A is down 45%; potassium is down 60%, and magnesium is down 85%

Cauliflower - Vitamin C is down 45%, Vitamin B1 is down 48%, and Vitamin B2 is down 47%

This is due to the lack of fertile soil and lack of nutrients (minerals) in the soil today.

If you've ever traveled overseas, you'll see a difference in the food – the size, the taste, etc.

Fiber

Fiber is another of the key ingredients to keeping you healthy and helping you lose weight. Fiber acts as the scrubbing bubbles that cleans your colon as it moves through your digestive tract. Fiber also acts as a prebiotic that allows your probiotics to work effectively. What is fiber, exactly? There is soluble fiber and insoluble fiber. Both are undigested. Fiber is considered a carbohydrate with no calories. Following is the difference between soluble and insoluble fiber according to the website www.healthcastle.com:

Insoluble Fiber

Functions of Insoluble Fiber

- move bulk through the intestines
- control and balance the pH (acidity) in the intestines

Benefits of Insoluble Fiber

- promote regular bowel movement and prevent constipation
- remove toxic waste through colon in less time

- help prevent colon cancer by keeping an optimal pH in intestines to prevent microbes from producing cancerous substances

Top Insoluble Fiber Foods

- Wheat bran, 11.3 grams of insoluble fiber per 1/2 cup
- All Bran cereal, 7.2 g per 1/3 cup
- Most beans (1/2 cup)
- Kidney beans, 5.9 g
- Pinto beans, 5.7 g
- Navy beans, 4.3 g
- Lentils, 4.6 g per 1/2 cup
- Shredded Wheat cereal, 4.5 g per cup
- Most Whole grains. Bulgur, for instance, contains 4.2 grams of insoluble fiber in 1/2 cup
- Flax seeds, 2.2 g per 1 tbsp
- Vegetables (1/2 cup)
- Okra, 3.1 g
- Turnip, 3.1 g
- Peas, 3 g

Soluble Fiber

Functions of Soluble Fiber

- they bind with fatty acids

- prolong stomach emptying time so that sugar is released and absorbed more slowly

Benefits of Soluble Fiber

- lower total cholesterol and LDL cholesterol (the Bad cholesterol) therefore reducing the risk of heart disease
- regulate blood sugar for people with diabetes

Top Soluble Fiber Foods

- Purple passion fruit, 6.5 g of soluble fiber per 1/2 cup
- Psyllium husk, 3.5 g per 1 Tbsp
- Metamucil, 3.4 g per 1 Tbsp
- Oat/Oat bran, 2.2 g per 3/4 cup
- Some Beans (1/2 cup)
- Black beans, 2.4 g
- Navy beans, 2.2 g
- Kidney beans, 2 g
- Soy
- Tofu, 2.8 g per 3/4 cup
- Edamame, 1.5 g per 1/2 cup
- Vegetables (1/2 cup)
- Avocado, 2.1 g
- Brussels sprouts, 2 g
- Sweet potato, 1.8 g

- Asparagus, 1.7 g

- Turnip, 1.7 g

- Fruit

- Dried figs, 1.9 g per 1/4 cup

- Orange, 1.8 g, medium size

- Fruit with skin, like pear, apricots, and nectarine, ~ 1.2 g

- Flax seed, 1.1 g per 1 tbsp

Fiber improves glucose tolerance, lowers cholesterol, and makes you feel full. Fiber slows down the digestive process. This is helpful because without fiber; carbs would get broken down into sucrose quickly which would cause an insulin response which, as we know, leads to fat storage and the inability to burn stored fats.

Water

Water is hugely important in both weight loss and general health. It is very important that you drink clean water that is free of chemicals and heavy metals. There are different types of water which are listed below.

Spring Water

Desalinated Water

Reverse Osmosis Water

Bottled Water

Filtered Water

Your body is approximately 60-70% water. If you lose 20% of your water content, you could die. That's how important it is to your health. Not drinking water can actually cause you to get fatter! Water assists your liver metabolize fat. Lack of water can decrease your physical performance.

Researchers at Loma Linda University said that people who drank five eight-ounce glasses of water daily were about half as likely to die of coronary heart disease as those who drank two glasses or less. Amazingly, drinking water appears to confer as much a benefit to heart health "as stopping smoking or lowering cholesterol," said Dr. Jacqueline Chan, who lead the study. (Fitness: The Complete Guide, Frederick Hatfield, PhD)

The common rule is that by the time you feel thirsty, you are already dehydrated. How much water should you drink every day? There is no hard and fast rule, because everyone is different. Some doctors say you should drink 8 glasses (8oz) of water per day. That's 64 ounces. Some say you should drink 16 ounces for every pound of weight lost during a workout. Other people have suggested 1 ounce per pound of body weight.

Dehydration has many detrimental effects on your body. According to Elaine Newkirk, ND, signs of dehydration include:

- Fatigue and weakness
- Anxiety
- Headaches
- Depression
- Constipation
- Cravings
- Intestinal cramps
- Heartburn
- Dry skin
- Dry mucous membranes of the nose, eyes, and throat
- Joint and back pain
- Nosebleeds
- Strong-smelling urine
- Migraines

- Colitis
- Nausea
- Low blood pressure
- Asthma and allergies
- Autoimmune diseases

Glycemic Index

The Glycemic Index is the measure of the ability that food has to raise our blood sugar. Glucose is the baseline set at 100, and all other foods are compared to that.

Following a low-glycemic index diet will allow you to keep your insulin response low, thus leading to the burning of fat. High-glycemic foods have a lot of sugar and can cause your body to produce insulin for as much as eighteen hours per day. And since insulin causes fat storage, that doesn't give your body much time to burn fat.

Let's take wheat as an example. Wheat comes in many forms. Fine white flour has the highest glycemic index followed by course flour, then cracked wheat, and lastly whole grain wheat. So, if you're going to eat wheat, you would want to avoid white flour and go with the whole grain. Keep in mind though, if you believe the information presented in Dr. Davis' book, Wheat Belly, then you may want to eliminate wheat from your diet entirely. I would highly suggest not eating wheat for a week or two and see the affect it has on your body. Generally speaking, the more a grain is processed, the higher it will rank on the glycemic index. So, a lot of your "healthy" breakfast cereals are actually very high on the glycemic index. For example, Total, Cheerios, Corn Flakes, and Puffed Wheat all have a glycemic index of 75. And Rice Krispies comes in at 80!

If you think you're being good to your body by eating low fat crackers, think again. Pretzels have a GI of 85. Corn Chips, Graham Crackers, and regular crackers have a GI of 75. Whole wheat crackers and Wheat Thins have a GI of 65. So, if you're snacking all day on crackers, you're putting yourself in a high insulin response mode all day long. Is it surprising you can't lose weight?!

I've put a Glycemic Index in the Appendix Section.

Chapter 12 - Super-foods

You should also fill your kitchen up with as many super-foods as you can. Super-foods can be broken down into various categories. The following list was taken from www.foodmatters.tv. They are an excellent resource. I highly recommend you visit their website.

Green Super-foods

Wheat grass

Wheat grass is the sprouted grass of a wheat seed. Unlike the whole grain, because it has been sprouted, it no longer contains gluten or other common allergic agents. Wheat grass is super alkalizing and is excellent for promoting healthy blood. It normalizes the thyroid gland to stimulate metabolism thus assisting digestion and promoting weight loss due also to its high enzyme content and cleansing effect.

According to www.wheatgrass.com, wheat grass has 40 positive effects on the body. A partial list includes:

- Best source of living chlorophyll
- High in oxygen
- Anti-bacterial
- Stops growth and development of unfriendly bacteria
- Rebuilds the bloodstream
- Detox agent
- Neutralizes toxins
- Purifies liver
- Improves blood sugar problems

Wheat grass is a natural source of vitamins and antioxidants, including:

Vitamins A, E, and B-12
Calcium
Selenium

Magnesium
Iron

One ounce of wheat grass juice is equal to the vitamin and mineral content of one ounce of fresh vegetables.

Barley grass

Barley grass has 11 times more calcium than cows' milk, 5 times more iron than spinach and 7 times more Vitamin C and bio-flavonoids than orange juice. It contains significant amounts of Vitamin B12 which is very important in a vegetarian diet. Barley grass juice has anti-viral activities and neutralizes heavy metals such as mercury in the blood.

Wild blue-green algae

Algae was the first form of life on Earth and its power is immense. Wild blue-green algae is a phyto-plankton and contains virtually every nutrient. With a 60% protein content and a more complete amino acid profile than beef or soy beans. It contains one of the best known food sources of beta carotene, B vitamins and chlorophyll. It has been shown to improve brain function and memory, strengthen the immune system and help with viruses, colds and flu.

Spirulina

Spirulina is a cultivated micro-algae which has been consumed for thousands of years by the indigenous peoples in MexicoN and Africa. It is one of the highest known protein sources on Earth and contains 70% complete protein, towering over steak which consists of only 25% protein once cooked. Studies have shown that spirulina can help control blood sugar levels and cravings thus making it a key food for diabetics, and can be used to assist in weight loss and as a general nutritional supplement.

Chlorella

Chlorella is a fresh water algae and like its other algae cousins contains a complete protein profile, all the B vitamins, vitamin C and E and many minerals. It is amazing for the immune system and for reducing cholesterol and preventing the hardening of the arteries, a precursor to heart attacks and strokes.

Fruit and Nut Super-foods

Fruit and nut super-foods are high in anti-oxidants that fight free radicals in the body. Free radicals may sound a little like an extremist terrorist sect evading capture and wreaking havoc across the globe and in fact within the context of your body this would be right. They are, in part, a natural occurrence through metabolism however extra and unnecessary free radical load can be put on our bodies by external factors including pollution, cigarette smoke, radiation, burnt foods, deep fried fats and cooked foods. When enough of these free radicals invade our immune system problems occurs. This is when you need antioxidants to build up the immune system and fight off the free radicals in the form of super-foods or supplements.

Goji Berries

Goji berries are grown on vines in the protected valleys of inner Mongolia and Tibet. These distinctively flavored red berries are a very rich source of vitamin C, having 500 times more vitamin C per ounce than oranges and actually more than any other fruit. They are a superb source of vitamins A, B1, B2, B6 and E and contain a full complement of protein with 18 amino acids and 21 trace minerals. Most of all they are an excellent antioxidant making it an ideal natural whole food for reversing aging and protecting against disease.

Raw Cacao

For this nut we could easily dedicate a whole page, if not a book. A word of warning before we start however, most cocoa powder and commercial chocolate is processed via the "Dutch method" meaning it is subjected to scorching temperatures of up to 150°C with the additional aid of solvents, thus destroying most of the nutrients and antioxidants. Be sure to attain certified organic raw cacao in a powder, nib or whole bean form as the temperature will have never been allowed to exceed 40°C thus allowing all the heat-sensitive vitamins, minerals and antioxidants to remain intact. Raw cacao beans contain possibly the world's most concentrated source of antioxidants found in any food. They are also extremely high in magnesium which has been found to be the most common deficient major mineral even following a balanced diet. For those concerned with not getting enough iron it should be pleasing to know that each serving of raw cacao beans contains 21% of the recommended daily allowance of iron. And if that is not enough raw cacao beans have an antioxidant (ORAC) score of 95,500. To put that into perspective, that is 14 times more flavonoids (antioxidants) than red wine and 21 times more than green tea.

Maca

Maca powder is from the Maca root, a flavorful ancient super-food from Peru. Maca has been cultivated for at least 2000 years and was consumed by Inca warriors to increase strength and endurance. It is a highly nutritious food that has been used traditionally to gain energy, promote sexual desire, support fertility and enhance immune system function. It continues today to be a significant staple food and medicinal plant for the Peruvian people and is now widely available around the world as a whole food supplement.

Acai

Acai berries have long been a part of the staple diet of the tribes in the Amazon. With the appearance of a purple grape and taste of a tropical berry it has been shown to have powerful antioxidant properties thanks to a high level of anthocyanins, pigments also found in red wine. The ORAC rating of acai is 1,027. Make sure to look for the freeze dried acai fruit in which the nutrients are kept intact or when buying the juice look for a brand that has not been pasteurized or heated in any way.

Coconuts

Young coconuts are one of the highest sources of electrolytes in nature. Electrolytes are ionized salts in our cells that transport energy throughout the body. Coconut water is a much better alternative to commercial sports drinks laden with artificial sugars and colors. The molecular structure of coconut water is identical to human blood plasma, which means that it is immediately recognized by the body and put to good use. Drinking the juice from a young coconut is like giving your body an instant blood transfusion. In fact this was common practice during World War II in the Pacific, where both sides in the conflict regularly used coconut water, siphoned directly from the coconut, to give emergency transfusions to wounded soldiers.

Coconut oil

Coconut oil's saturated fat is of the medium-chain fatty acid variety, which are digested more easily and utilized differently by the body than other saturated fats (such as butter, meat and eggs). Whereas other saturated fats are stored in the body's cells, the medium chain fatty acids in coconut oil are sent directly to the liver where they are immediately converted into energy. Coconut oil will actually speed up metabolism so your body will burn more calories in a day which will contribute to weight loss. Coconut oil supports healthy metabolic function and is a revered anti-bacterial, anti-viral and anti-fungal agent. Pacific islanders deem coconut oil to be the cure-all gift from nature for all illness.

Noni

This fruit has been used by Polynesian islanders as a regenerative medicine for more than 1500 years. Research documents that the noni fruit has astounding anti-bacterial properties, even against E-coli. It has anti-tumor activity, anti-inflammatory properties, is effective as a pain reliever, generates cell repair and strengthens the immune system. Noni contains a multitude of vitamins, minerals, enzymes and phytonutrients. Many believe that the synergistic effect of the multi-spectrum nutrients is what gives it its potency. It has been proven beneficial for colds and flu's, digestive disorders, skin disorders, pain relief, headaches, infections and more. For best results look for a freeze-dried product that uses only the whole fruit or when buying the juice look for a brand that does not use pasteurizing.

Bee Super-foods

Royal Jelly

Royal Jelly is a milk like secretion from the head glands of the worker bees. The queen bee lives almost exclusively on royal jelly and she lives around 40 times longer than the rest of the bees. Royal Jelly is a powerhouse of nutrients containing every nutrient necessary to support life. It is the world's richest source of pantothenic acid (also known as Vitamin B5), which is known to combat stress, fatigue and insomnia and is a vital nutrient for healthy skin and hair.

Bee Pollen

Bee pollen is collected by bees from flowering plants and formed into granules. Bee pollen is the most complete food found in nature and has five to seven times more protein than beef. It is especially beneficial for the extra nutritional and energy needs of athletes and those recovering from illness. It is a natural antidote for fighting allergies particularly hay fever and sinusitis. Research shows that bee pollen counteracts the signs of aging and increases both mental and physical capability.

Propolis

Propolis is the substance that bees coat the walls of their hives with and bee hives have often been referred to as the most antiseptic places in nature. The powerful antibiotic properties of propolis can help protect humans from bacteria and can strengthen our immune system. Propolis works against viruses, something that antibiotics cannot do. Research shows that taking propolis during the high risk 'cold and flu' season reduces colds, coughing and inflammation of the mouth, tonsils and throat.

Seaweed Superfoods

Benefits of Seaweeds

Blood Purifying: The chemical composition of seaweeds is so close to human blood plasma, that they are excellent at regulating and purifying our blood.

High in Calcium: They can contain up to 10 times more calcium than milk and 8 times as much as beef.

Alkalizing: They help to alkalize our blood, neutralizing the over-acidic effects of our modern diet.

Have Powerful Chelating Properties: They offer protection from a wide array of environmental toxins, including heavy metals, pollutants and radiation by-products, by converting them to harmless salts that the body can eliminate easily.

Contain Anti-oxidants: Seaweeds contain lignans (naturally occurring chemical compounds) which have anti-cancer properties.

Detoxifying: They are rich in chlorophyll (the pigment that makes some seaweeds green) which is a powerful, natural detoxifier that helps to draw out waste products.

Boost Weight loss: Seaweeds play a role in boosting weight loss and deterring cellulite build-up. Their naturally high concentration of iodine, helps to stimulate the thyroid gland, which is responsible for maintaining a healthy metabolism. At the same time, its' minerals act like electrolytes to break the chemical bonds that seal the fat cells, allowing trapped wastes to escape.

Seaweeds

Nori

Nori is best known as the seaweed used to make sushi rolls. You can make your own at home, but make sure you use the untoasted nori sheets for maximum nutrient content.

Kelp

Kelp, also known as brown algae, is the most common seaweed found along the ocean shores. Due to its thick leaves it is perfect for a hot seaweed bath. It is also available in supplement form.

Dulse

Dulse is a red seaweed and can be bought either whole or as flakes. Dulse sold as flakes does not need to be soaked and can be added straight to any meal. Whole dulse is better soaked, drained of water, and sliced before adding to your dish. It is great to use as seasoning on salads, vegetables and soups.

Arame

Arame is a 'black' stringy looking seaweed. It needs to be soaked for a few minutes before it is added to cooking, where it will double in size. It can be added to any grain dishes, stir fries, soups, salads and curries.

Wakame

A deep green seaweed, wakame is sold fresh or dehydrated. It tastes best when hydrated in water for a few minutes before being used. Sprinkle in soups, stocks, stews, stir fries or savory dishes.

Kombu

Used in Japan for centuries as a mineral rich flavor enhancer. Add a strip of kombu when cooking beans to make them more digestible and to reduce gas. Add a strip of kombu to your sprouts when soaking them to allow them to soak up the minerals.

When sourcing or buying seaweed, choose certified organic brands where possible. Seaweeds will absorb the properties of the water in which they are grown, so you want to ensure that they have been grown and harvested in unpolluted waters that are pure, and free from harmful chemicals.

Herb Super-foods

Nettle

The bowel mover. These plants are best known as stinging nettle plants. However, when the nettle leaves are dried and eaten, the saliva is able to neutralize the sting. Nettles are incredibly effective in removing unwanted pounds. A cup of nettle tea in the morning is ideal to get things going in the bowel department. The nettle leaves increase the thyroid function, increase metabolism and releases mucus in the colon allowing for the flushing of excess wastes.

Aloe vera

Aloe vera is a perennial succulent that grows in a wild and seems to do best in tropical and sub-tropical areas. It has been deemed a super-food after research studies identifying its seventy-five healing compounds including natural steroids, antibiotic agents, amino acids, minerals and enzymes. Aloe vera has been used since Egyptian times as a skin moisturizer, and healer for burns, cuts, bruises, acne and eczema. This is mostly due to the high concentration of natural sulphur (MSM) that it contains. Aloe juices alkalizes the digestive tract preventing over-acidity, a common cause of indigestion, acid reflux, heartburn and ulcers.

Echinacea

Echinacea is a household name when it comes to warding off colds and flu. This herb is used as a natural antibiotic and immune system stimulator, helping to build up resistance. The reason for its effectiveness is because of its ability to stimulate the lymph flow in the body. Lymph runs parallel with our bloodstream and carries toxins out of the body. The herb can be taken in liquid or capsule form for 2-3 week periods during "high risk" flu seasons. The tea from this herb has also grown in popularity for treating infections and cancers including skin cancer.

Ginseng

Ginseng is the quintessential herb for handling stress. This ancient healing herb has been used widely throughout Asia as an energizer tonic. This special herb is particularly beneficial when recovering from illness or surgery for its restorative and anti-infection properties. It promotes regeneration from stress and fatigue.

(www.foodmatters.tv)

Chapter 13 – Exercise

Of course, we can't forget about exercise. Exercise is half the process involved in losing weight and being healthy. So, fifty percent is diet and fifty percent is exercise. Doing either will have results, but it won't give you the optimum results that you might be looking for. If you eat right but don't exercise, you'll still be flabby. You want your muscles to be toned and buff. Muscles increase your resting metabolic rate, so by having muscles, you'll be burning more calories. There are different types of exercise with different results. There is resistance training and there is cardiovascular training. You can train for strength, power, agility, speed, etc. You can train to be lean or you can train to bulk up.

Now, I talk to women all the time who don't like to work out because they don't want to look like a body builder and they don't want to "bulk up". Let me assure you, it takes a lot of effort (probably more than you're willing to put in) for a woman to bulk up like a body builder. Trust me, when you shed those excess pounds, you want to have some lean muscles underneath with good definition to show off. So if you're worried about getting bulky, don't worry about it.

"How much and what kind of exercise should I be doing?"

There are so many different kinds of exercises. You can go with no weights, just using your body weight. You can use dumbbells. You can use kettle bells. You can use various types of free weights. You can use bands. You can use machines. You can use stability balls or medicine balls. You can do step classes, cardio classes, spinning, kick boxing, yoga, tai chi, chi gong, etc. It really depends on what you like to do and what kind of equipment you have access to.

Will you be working out at home or at the gym? You'll see some people working out in the gym for hours. Personally, I think that's unnecessary. Doctors nowadays say that 30-60 minutes per day is what you need. Some people do 30 minutes of cardio and then do weights. Some people do weights and then do cardio. I personally like to combine the two and do a fast-paced workout that works multiple body parts at once while also ramping up my cardio. I can squeeze a 60-90 minute workout into 30-40 minutes. But it will kick your butt.

In general, good health can be achieved by:

Food = 50%

Exercise = 50%

    Resistance Training = 25%

    Cardio Training = 25%

Aerobics and Cardiovascular Training

Cardiovascular training is good for your heart, your waistline, and your overall health. Some examples of cardio training include running, swimming, cycling, rowing, treadmills, stair climbers, and cross-training. When it comes to losing weight, aerobics is an important part of your workout routine. But, like anything else, too much is not good. Aerobics can burn as much as 1000 calories per hour. But too much aerobics can cause free radical damage. So, like everything else, moderation is key. On the positive side, aerobics can increase your energy, relieve depression, relieve stress, reduce the risk of heart disease, increase HDL (good cholesterol), lower blood pressure, improve sleep, and increase your mental capacity.

Heart Rate

What is your resting heart rate? When you wake up in the morning, take your pulse. Count the number of beats in six seconds, then multiply that number by ten. That is your resting heart rate. Typically, the healthier you are, the lower your heart rate will be. Of course, a heart rate that is too low is not good, but in general, if your resting heart rate is between 60-70 beats per minute, you're doing okay. If your heart rate is up around 90-100, you may want to visit your doctor and get checked out. What should your heart rate be when working out? Although everyone is different, people generally use the formula 220 – your age x 75%. Your maximum heart rate is 220 – your age. Then take seventy-five percent of that number. I suggest buying a heart rate monitor to keep track of your heart rate while working out.

How much aerobic training do you need? It should be sufficient to do a thirty-minute workout, three to four days per week. If you are doing aerobics forty-five minutes per day for over four days a week, it may not be doing yourself any extra good. The goal of aerobics is not, as some think, to raise your heart rate. Rather, the goal of aerobics is to raise and maintain a higher level of metabolism.

Resistance Training

The following is a comparison between machines and free weights. This list comes from Fitness: The Complete Guide by Frederick Hatfield, PhD. It is a good list.

Advantages of Free Weights:

- *Dumbbells and barbells are more effective in developing the smaller synergistic (helping muscles) and stabilizer muscles.*

- *Free weight exercises more closely match the neurological patterns of associated sports skills from a biomechanical point of view, because of joint kinesthesis, leverage similarities, and bodily involvement.*

- *Barbells and dumbbells are more versatile.*

- *Barbells and dumbbells are less expensive.*

- *Barbells and dumbbells take up less space.*

- Greater overall strength can be achieved using barbells and dumbbells.

- Power is improved more efficiently and to a greater extent through the use of free weights.

- Other aspects of fitness, including size, flexibility, reduced body fat, and muscle toning are achieved more efficiently through the use of free weights.

Disadvantages of Free Weights:

- Barbells and dumbbells that are adjustable can come apart if care is not taken to tightly secure the collars.

- Adjustments in weight from set to set requires affixing or removing plates and replacing and removing collars – often a time-consuming and tedious ordeal.

- You need large spaces to use barbells and dumbbells; it can be hazardous for large groups of unorganized people to use them in a small area.

- In certain exercises, it is difficult, if not impossible, to derive maximum isolation of a muscle or muscle group.

Advantages of Machines:

- Some machines are more efficient in isolating muscle or muscle group for more efficient overload.

- For group use, some machines are more efficient in terms of space utilization (especially Universal machines).

- Machines are easier to use, and therefore faster workouts are possible. Less time is usually wasted changing pates and waiting for spotters.

Disadvantages of Machines:

- *All machines are not alike, but most require the moving of a weight along a predetermined path (or track), making it nearly impossible to derive synergistic or stabilizer muscle strength.*

- *Machines that control movement velocity (such as isokinetic machines) or vary the resistance over a given movement (such as Nautilus or Universal machines) have removed the "natural" aspect from the exercise. Many physiologists claim this renders such machines less effective in developing strength and size citing differing neurological input as the chief reason.*

- *Because of machine construction constraints, it is generally impossible to achieve maximum velocity, and high-speed training is often a prerequisite in sports training. The machines may break, jerk about violently, or simply not accommodate such training.*

- *Most machines are built to serve the average-sized person. Very short or very tall people find it almost impossible to use many of the machines currently on the market.*

- *Machines tend to be in a price range beyond the means of many gym owners, and often beyond the means of commercial spas as well.*

- *Many machines are so specialized that one would have to purchase several in order to get even a marginally effective workout, floor space and budget permitting.*

- *The space-age appearance of many machines lulls users into believing that high technology equals maximum efficiency in achieving fitness goals, a sentiment that is definitely not true. Nothing beats hard work.*

- *The cam designs on variable resistance machines are frequently (more often than not) inaccurate; that is, they do not conform to the force curve of the intended movement. Thus, far less benefit is derived from its use than you would expect from free weights.*

If you want to see some of my workout routines, I have videos available on my website and I sell workout DVDs, as well. I also am in the middle of writing a workout book you can purchase.

Of course, exercise will help you lose weight, but did you know that while you're exercising to lose weight, you're also reducing your risk of disease? According to Dr. Kulkarni,

"Research has shown that exercise helps with sleep disorders, reduces risk of cancer and cardiovascular disease, reduces cholesterol and triglycerides, can provide the benefits of hormone-replacement therapy (without the side-effects) for menopausal women, can help reduce fibroids, helps some with chronic fatigue, can help with arthritis pain, can help those with lupus, can increase natural killer cells (improves the immune system) reduces stress, helps with obesity, increases life span, and more."

I highly suggest hiring a Personal Trainer to help you with your weight-loss goals. There really is a lot of information behind fitness training that most people don't know about. For example, there have been books written about each of the chapters I have in this book. The book I studied to become a Personal Trainer was over 700-pages long. So when you decide to start working out, create a budget for a Personal Trainer, if you can. At least for a month or two. If you want to see results, spend the money and do it right.

For example, do you just go in and work out or do you warm up first? Do you know the benefits of warming up? Do you know the benefits of cooling down? Do you know how different grips affect the exercise? Do you know how to breathe correctly? Do you know what you should or shouldn't eat before and after a workout? Do you know how to calculate your daily caloric intake? The reason people don't normally get good results is because they just think if they go to the gym and workout, they'll get results. Not true. I see people at the gym all the time who are doing exercises incorrectly. I've seen people going to the gym for months without achieving any results. It's really unfortunate and unnecessary. And, of course, there are a lot of ideas floating around out there that people believe that are simply untrue.

Fact vs. Fiction

Just like we discussed facts and labeling, there are some myths in the fitness industry and I want to clarify.

"All you need is aerobics to lose weight"

The thinking comes from the "calories in calories out" club. Assuming you burn more calories while running on the treadmill than you consume during the day. But just doing aerobics doesn't preserve lean muscle mass. The less lean muscle you have, the lower your metabolism. Remember that it takes more energy to sustain muscle than fat, so by building muscle, you will be burning more calories. Aerobics does not build lean muscle. My suggestion would be to do both aerobics and weight training to lose weight.

"You lose more fat the more you sweat"

Any weight lost from sweating is probably just water weight. Some people sweat more than others, but sweating is typically dependent on such things as body temperature, room temperature, humidity, amount of physical conditioning, and body composition. On the other hand, sweating is one of the ways your body detoxifies, so sweating is definitely a good thing.

"You can burn fat from specific areas of your body"

You'll hear commercials on TV saying that if you take their supplement, it will burn belly fat. Or if you do sit-ups you will burn the fat around your stomach. This is simply not true. What will decrease the size of your belly is taking enzymes and probiotics while decreasing your carbs, but not from any specific exercise.

"Drinking milk and dairy products causes cellulite"

Cellulite is caused more from genetics. Cellulite can be decreased with deep massage. Some people also use body brushing to remove cellulite. You may want to try either of those. On the other hand, drinking milk can cause a mucus buildup in your system and lead to allergies and other problems.

"When you stop working out, muscles turn to fat"

Completely untrue. Muscles are muscles and fat is fat. Muscles cannot turn into fat. It's like saying your goldfish can turn into a puppy. If you don't use your muscles, they will atrophy and become smaller. At the same time, you will gain more fat, so as your muscles decrease, your fat increases.

"You burn more fat doing aerobics at a lower intensity"

According to *Fitness: The Complete Guide*, "The absolute amount of fat calories burned during high-intensity exercise tends to be equal to or greater than the number burned during low-intensity exercise, even though the percentage of calories burned from fat is higher during low–intensity exercise." There are a lot of other factors involved in burning fat including the food you eat and if you're also doing weight training.

Chapter 14 – Supplements

Although we covered vitamins and minerals earlier, I want to go over other types of supplements that some people use in their diet and exercise routine. There are thousands of supplements on the market today. Some of these supplements may be worthwhile, while others are not. I want to write a little about these supplements to show how things change with time and how you may not want to get caught up in the hype of every new supplement that comes along. Of course, you should check with your health care professional before jumping into supplements. Generally speaking, I would keep my supplements to a minimum and stick with eating healthy first.

Creatine

Studies have shown that creatine can improve strength performance and increase lean body mass. It seems to work equally well with both men and women in increasing high intensity exercise performance ability. As mentioned earlier, as you build muscle, you will burn more fat, simply because it takes more energy to maintain muscle.

Ephedrine

On the positive side, ephedrine speeds up your metabolism. It causes your body to release adrenaline. Adrenaline, in turn, causes the release of glucose from the liver. It also helps break down fatty acids in your body. Ephedrine is typically combined with caffeine for weight-loss programs.

On the negative side, there are a number of issues with Ephedrine, and supplements containing Ephedrine. It has been shown to cause high blood pressure, irregular heart rate, insomnia, nervousness, tremors, headaches, seizures, heart attacks, strokes, and death. Needless to say, I would not recommend it.

Conjugated Linoleic Acid (CLA)

CLA is a free fatty acid as well as an antioxidant, anti-carcinogen, and anti-catabolite that is made by the breakdown of linoleic acid (Omega-6). It blocks carcinogens, inhibits the storage of fats, and increases the breakdown of fats. It may increase metabolism, enhance muscle growth, and lower insulin resistance. It is found naturally in free-range meat, dairy, corn oil, and sunflower oil.

Chromium

Chromium is a mineral that can be found in food. It is used often in weight loss programs, because it works with insulin in carb, fat, and protein metabolism. Chromium is typically found in the form of Chromium Piccolinate. Some of the best sources of chromium in your diet would be broccoli and grape juice (fresh, not processed.) Chromium is measured in micrograms, so you don't need much. An adult woman needs approximately 25 mcg per day. An adult male needs approximately 35 mcg per day.

DHEA

DHEA is a steroid hormone produced primarily by the adrenal glands. In some studies, it was shown to increase fat metabolism without increasing testosterone levels. Other studies didn't show any results with regard to weight loss but did seem to improve mood, immune system enhancement, and acted as an anti-depressant. On the downside, nobody should take DHEA if you have prostate issues (men) or if you have a tendency toward breast cancer or reproductive cancer (women).

Androstendione

"Andro" use was extremely popular in gyms for guys (and girls) who wanted to get pumped up. Testing has not shown any significant increase in strength or testosterone levels, but it is still popular among gym-goers. I don't recommend it.

Ribose

Ribose is used in the production of ATP which creates energy in the body. It helps heart cells and muscle cells maintain their energy. Your workout effectiveness can be increased by taking Ribose before, during, and after a workout. Ribose has been deemed safe, and tests have shown no lasting side effects. If you take too much, you could get diarrhea or mild hypoglycemia.

Carnitine

Carnitine can reduce your risk of coronary heart disease by improving blood flow, raising good cholesterol (HDL) and lowering bad cholesterol (LDL). It can increase your metabolic rate and can help in fat metabolism by transporting fat into the mitochondria thus increasing the rate at which your body uses fat for energy. There is some controversy about how much carnitine actually helps with weight loss.

CoQ10

CoQ10 is a co-enzyme and fat-soluble antioxidant that is beneficial for the heart, gums, and varicose veins. It lowers your resting heart rate and increases endurance. It has the ability to generate cellular energy and boost metabolism. It also helps to regulate the fats and sugars in your blood. I recommend it for weight loss and heart health.

SAMe

SAMe comes from the amino acid methionine and plays an important role in many biochemical processes in your body that keep you healthy. Your body produces SAMe, but if it doesn't produce enough, it could lead to degenerative diseases. SAMe is involved with many body biochemical functions including: DNA function, manufacture of proteins; liver function; fat metabolism; the production of nervous system and brain biochemical such as ephedrine and dopamine; fetal development; hormone regulation; cell membrane integrity; cell reproduction; and brain and nervous system function. (Fitness, The Complete Guide, Fredrick C. Hatfield, PhD)

Glucosamine

For people who are going to be working out a lot in order to build muscle and reduce fat, glucosamine is helpful in the rebuilding of connective tissue. It reduces pain, stiffness, and joint mobility. You may see Glucosamine combined with Chondroitin in pill form for joint relief.

Protein Powder

There are different types of protein powder on the market today. Whey protein comes from milk production, so if you are lactose intolerant, whey protein may not be the right choice for you. Whey protein will help build your muscle, increases your physical performance, improve your circulation, and has potential anti-aging effects. Check the labels and make sure your protein is not full of fillers. Other protein powders are made from eggs white, soy, pea, and hemp. Take a look at Jay Robb's protein. It's good quality. I recommend protein shakes.

Glutamine

Glutamine is a "non-essential" amino acid. Your body produces glutamine, and sixty percent of it is kept in your muscles. The other forty percent is found in the tissue of your lung, liver, brain, and stomach. The harder you train, the more glutamine your body releases. Over-training may cause a depletion of glutamine. It buffers poisonous waste such as ammonia. Glutamine is needed to make DNA. According to Ronald Klatz, MD, President of the Academy of Anti-Aging Medicine in Chicago, *"Glutamine promotes the assimilation of nutrients, regulates protein synthesis, stimulates growth-hormone production and enhances the immune system."* *(Fitness, The Complete Guide, Fredrick C. Hatfield, PhD)*. Therefore, you want to have enough glutamine in your system.

Garcinia Cambogia / Hydroxycitric Acid

HCA is the main ingredient in Garcinia Cambogia which has been around for quite some time but recently made popular again by Dr. Oz. It helps burn fat in the mitochondria and amplifies satiety through the vagus nerve to the brain.

Lecithin

Not only does lecithin improve digestion, but it has a list of benefits including improving brain function, boosting immune system, and reducing cholesterol. It also helps skin conditions, prevents vitamin deficiencies, and loosens blood clots. Lecithin can be found in organ meats, grain, salad oil, seeds and nuts, and egg yolks. (That's right folks – yolks!)

Branch Chain Amino Acids

You may have noticed nutrition companies promoting Branch Chain Amino Acids. There are three – leucine, isoleucine, and valine. BCAA's comprise about 35% of the amino acid content in your muscles. Leucine is used at twice the rate as the other two, so you may see a higher amount of leucine in your BCAA supplement. BCAA's can increase your lean body mass and give you more strength.

Liquid Ionic Minerals

Liquid minerals are better absorbed than minerals in tablet form, and natural, plant-derived, organic liquid minerals are the best. Minerals in tablet form and synthetic minerals are only absorbed about 20%. Quality minerals are typically plant-derived, contain Fulvic Acid, stay "in solution", are produced using purified water, and are natural. Poor quality minerals come from sea water, come from inorganic sources, don't have Fulvic Acid, and are produced using hydrochloric acid.

Desiccated Liver

Desiccated means that liver (typically from beef) is dried and powdered. Liver is high in B-Vitamins (B12 and folic acid), iron, protein, and copper. It has the ability to increase recovery from your exercise. Desiccated liver is used by people who work out a lot to increase energy and stamina.

The following list comes from Fitness: the Complete Guide by Frederick Hatfield, PhD

To Lose Fat, take:

- *DHEA*
- *Energy Drinks (long-chain glucose polymers)*
- *Meal Replacement Drinks (with balanced micro and macro-nutrients from high grade sources*
- *Herbal Formulas (xaio pangmei, brindall berry, qing herb formulas)*
- *Coffee (caffeine)*
- *Yerba Mate (stereo-isomer of caffeine)*
- *Bifidobacteria*
- *Alpha ketoisocaproate (KIC)*
- *Other lipotropic substances*

To get stronger, take:

- *Protein drinks with egg or whey*
- *Ornithine alphaketoglutarate (OKG)*
- *Branched Chain Amino Acids (BCAAs)*
- *Insulin-like growth factors (colostrum)*
- *L-Glutamine*
- *Herbal Formulas*
- *Alpha ketoisocaproate (KIC)*

To build muscle mass, take:

- *Creatine Monohydrate*
- *Protein Drinks with egg or whey*
- *Ornithine alphadetoglutarate (OKG)*
- *Branch Chain Amino Acids (BCAAs)*
- *Medium-Chain Triglycerides (MCT oil)*
- *Insulin-like Growth Factors (colostrum)*
- *L-Glutamine*
- *Herbal Formulas*
- *Flaxseed Oil*
- *Arginine*

For General Health, take:

- *Vitamin and Mineral Complex*
- *Antioxidants (Vitamins A, C, and E, glutathione, selenium, green tea, ginko biloba)*
- *Trace Elements*
- *Immune Boosters (colostrum, mumie, Echinacea, DHEA)*
- *Individual Amino Acids*
- *Chaparral, maria thistle, anthocyanadins*
- *Cardiovascular Tonics (garlic, onion, ginger, cayenne, skullcap, black cohash, goldenseal, valerian, hawthorn berries)*
- *Adaptogens (Siberian Ginseng)*
- *Bifidobacteria*

Chapter 15 – Body Systems, Hormones, Glands, Genetics

I want to take a little time to discuss some of the body systems, hormones, glands, and genetics, because people always have questions about it.

Genetics

Let's begin with genetics. People will claim that the reason they are fat is because it's their genetics. Horse hockey! Yes, we all have our own set of genetics, but I hate using genetics as an excuse, because it's a cop out. Don't buy into that argument. Your genetics may give you a different body type and it may cause your body to process nutrients differently, but you are probably not overweight because of your genes. Here's another test. Look at people (and your own family) over that past 100 years. Are your parents fat? Maybe. Are your grandparents fat? Were your great-grandparents fat? Has everyone in your family for the past 100 years been fat? I highly doubt it. If you are genetically predisposed to being fat, then everyone in your family throughout history would also have those same genes. With proper nutrition and exercise, you can reduce your body fat percentage. You may not look like your skinny neighbor who has a different body type, but for your own body type, you can be less fat. The food you eat and the lifestyle you live can affect your genes, though. So, you can change your genes which will have an effect on your own children.

Let me give you an example of what I'm talking about. A survey by the American Institute for Cancer Research showed that eighty-six percent of the people they surveyed thought that genes cause cancer when, in reality, only about ten to fifteen percent of cancer is caused by genetics. (The rest are caused by environmental factors and lifestyle.)

(Food as Medicine, Dr. Dharma Singh Khalsa, M.D.)

Body Systems

Your body has twelve systems:

1. Skeletal
2. Muscular
3. Cardiovascular
4. Lymphatic
5. Nervous
6. Endocrine
7. Integument (skin)
8. Respiratory
9. Digestive
10. Urinary
11. Immune
12. Reproductive

They are all important, but the ones that deal more with your weight issues are the Digestive System, your Endocrine System, your Cardiovascular System, and your Muscular System. When discussing detoxification, we also talk about the Lymph, Skin, Respiratory, and Urinary Systems. This book has focused primarily on the Digestive and Muscular Systems for a reason. Your endocrine system is key in keeping you healthy and helping you lose weight, but eating right, digesting right, and exercising can control your endocrine system and your body will operate the way it is supposed to.

Your endocrine system works on hormones and glands. Are hormones important for health and weight loss? Absolutely. Do your glands control your hormones? Yes. But what controls your glands? The nutrients you absorb from your food. The problem in today's world is that we treat the symptoms rather than going to the source of the problem. For example, you might hear that a person is overweight because they have an under active thyroid gland. This is a true statement. Your thyroid controls your metabolism. But leaving it there is too simplistic. You may know that your thyroid needs iodine to function correctly. But did you know that in order for your body to absorb and utilize iodine, you also need vitamin A, Vitamin E, Zinc, Iron, fat, and protein? Did you know that sugar, caffeine, fluorine, fluoride, bromine, and chlorine make it difficult for your body to absorb iodine? So, you can see that even though your thyroid may not be functioning correctly, it may not be genetics and it may be fixable through making corrections in your diet. And where does your body get iodine? You can get it from kelp, bladder-wrack, and Siberian ginseng, or you can take an iodine tincture. By the way, when I say that the thyroid needs vitamin A and E, Zinc, Iron, fat and protein to absorb iodine, it means that your body has to be able to ABSORB those nutrients. Continuing the same thinking, in order to absorb protein, for example, your body needs hydrochloric acid, pepsin, and protease (enzymes). In order to absorb vitamin A, your body needs zinc, protein, essential fatty acids, bile, lipase, and probiotics. That circles us back around to the digestive system. Are you beginning to see that everything comes back to digestion and absorption? If you are not absorbing nutrients (even if you are taking them) then you won't be getting the results you want.

My point is that your body is a very complex piece of machinery. You can get deep into the weeds if you try to treat every little symptom that comes up. We can make health very complicated, or we can make it simple. We can get into the chemistry and molecular structure or we can just start living a more healthy and natural lifestyle. Don't let your doctor or anybody else make your health so complicated that you just give up.

Chapter 16 – Other Holistic Approaches

Massage

The Physical Benefits of Massage Therapy

- relaxes the body
- quiets the mind
- calms the nervous system
- lowers blood pressure
- reduces heart rate
- slows respiration
- stretches connective tissue
- loosens tight muscles
- reduces chronic pain
- improves skin tone
- increases blood and lymph circulation
- relieves tired and aching muscles
- stimulates the release of endorphins
- improves muscle tone
- relieves cramps and muscle spasms
- increases flexibility
- promotes deeper more effective breathing
- strengthens the immune system
- reduces swelling
- breaks up scar and adipose tissue (fat tissue)
- increases metabolism
- decreases muscular deterioration
- increases oxygen to the brain
- assists in eliminating toxins from the body
- increases range of motion and flexibility

Massage should be a part of your overall wellness program. It may not directly cause weight loss, but by working on various body systems, it is a great adjunct to diet and exercise.

Herbology

There are many herbs that are used not only for weight-loss programs but also for general health and specific ailments. Herbs that are good for your metabolism and weight loss include:

Astragalus – Increases your metabolism

Bladderwrack – Increases you body's ability to burn fat and stimulates your thyroid

Cayenne Pepper – Increases your metabolism

Chickweed – Helps with fat metabolism

Coleus Forkskohlii – Stimulates lipolysis (fat breakdown).

Ashwagandha - Increases thyroid hormone production and reduces cortisol levels.

Garcinia Cambogia – Assists with fat metabolism

Ginger – Increases metabolism

Ginko – Effective against a slowing metabolism

Greet Tea – Increases you metabolism

Milk Thistle – Aids in liver detoxification and metabolism of carbs, fats, and protein

Panax Ginseng – When exercising, it shifts energy productions towards fatty acids

Sage – Decreases your appetite

Schizandra – Helps regulate blood sugar swings and stimulates metabolic functions

Siberian Ginseng - Acts to normalize blood sugar and helps regulate thyroid

Herbs that specifically help digestion include:

Milk Thistle	Goldenseal	Peppermint
Dandelion Root	Aloe	Ginger
Slippery Elm	Chamomile	Turmeric
Marshmallow	Wild Yam	Bayberry
Fennel	Licorice	Schizandra

Acupuncture

If you don't mind needles, acupuncture is another modality you can utilize for weight loss. I know acupuncturists who have been very successful working with people who need to lose weight. Acupuncture works with the energy pathways in your body and how it affects your internal organs.

Homeopathy

There are many homeopathic remedies that can help you lose weight. These remedies work on an energetic level to help your organs function more efficiently. Homeopathy works for many types of issues in addition to weight loss, so if you have other issues, you may want to visit a Homeopathic Doctor.

Meditation

Mediation has so many positive benefits that can help you not only to lose weight, but in many different aspects of your life. From the website www.IneedMotivation.com, we get a list of 100 benefits of meditation.

Physiological benefits:
1- It lowers oxygen consumption.
2- It decreases respiratory rate.
3- It increases blood flow and slows the heart rate.
4- Increases exercise tolerance.
5- Leads to a deeper level of physical relaxation.

6- Good for people with high blood pressure.
7- Reduces anxiety attacks by lowering the levels of blood lactate.
8- Decreases muscle tension
9- Helps in chronic diseases like allergies, arthritis etc.
10- Reduces Pre-menstrual Syndrome symptoms.
11- Helps in post-operative healing.
12- Enhances the immune system.
13- Reduces activity of viruses and emotional distress
14- Enhances energy, strength and vigor.
15- Helps with weight loss
16- Reduction of free radicals, less tissue damage
17- Higher skin resistance
18- Drop in cholesterol levels, lowers risk of cardiovascular disease.
19- Improved flow of air to the lungs resulting in easier breathing.
20- Decreases the aging process.
21- Higher levels of DHEAS (Dehydroepiandrosterone)
22- Prevented, slowed or controlled pain of chronic diseases
23- Makes you sweat less
24- Cure headaches & migraines
25- Greater Orderliness of Brain Functioning
26- Reduced Need for Medical Care
27- Less energy wasted
28- More inclined to sports, activities
29- Significant relief from asthma
30- Improved performance in athletic events
31- Normalizes to your ideal weight
32- Harmonizes our endocrine system
33- Relaxes our nervous system
34- Produce lasting beneficial changes in brain electrical activity
35- Cure infertility (the stresses of infertility can interfere with the release of hormones that regulate ovulation).

Psychological benefits:
36- Builds self-confidence.
37- Increases serotonin level, influences mood and behavior.
38- Resolve phobias & fears
39- Helps control own thoughts

40- Helps with focus & concentration
41- Increase creativity
42- Increased brain wave coherence.
43- Improved learning ability and memory.
44- Increased feelings of vitality and rejuvenation.
45- Increased emotional stability.
46- Improved relationships
47- Mind ages at slower rate
48- Easier to remove bad habits
49- Develops intuition
50- Increased Productivity
51- Improved relations at home & at work
52- Able to see the larger picture in a given situation
53- Helps ignore petty issues
54- Increased ability to solve complex problems
55- Purifies your character
56- Develop will power
57- Greater communication between the two brain hemispheres
58- React more quickly and more effectively to a stressful event.
59- Increases one's perceptual ability and motor performance
60- Higher intelligence growth rate
61- Increased job satisfaction
62- Increase in the capacity for intimate contact with loved ones
63- Decrease in potential mental illness
64- Better, more sociable behavior
65- Less aggressiveness
66- Helps in quitting smoking, alcohol addiction
67- Reduces need and dependency on drugs, pills & pharmaceuticals
68- Need less sleep to recover from sleep deprivation
69- Require less time to fall asleep, helps cure insomnia
70- Increases sense of responsibility
71- Reduces road rage
72- Decrease in restless thinking
73- Decreased tendency to worry
74- Increases listening skills and empathy
75- Helps make more accurate judgments

76- Greater tolerance

77- Gives composure to act in considered & constructive ways

78- Grows a stable, more balanced personality

79- Develops emotional maturity

Spiritual benefits:

80- Helps keep things in perspective

81- Provides peace of mind, happiness

82- Helps you discover your purpose

83- Increased self-actualization.

84- Increased compassion

85- Growing wisdom

86- Deeper understanding of yourself and others

87- Brings body, mind, spirit in harmony

88- Deeper Level of spiritual relaxation

89- Increased acceptance of oneself

90- Helps learn forgiveness

91- Changes attitude toward life

92- Creates a deeper relationship with your God

93- Attain enlightenment

94- Greater inner-directedness

95- Helps living in the present moment

96- Creates a widening, deepening capacity for love

97- Discovery of the power and consciousness beyond the ego

98- Experience an inner sense of "Assurance or Knowingness"

99- Experience a sense of "Oneness"

100- Increases the synchronicity in your life

Chapter 17 – The Solution: Suggestions for a Healthy Lifestyle

The Beginning

First, set aside a certain amount of money that you can use as your Health Fund. Don't think of adding it to your current monthly budget, but rather as a replacement cost. You will be decreasing the amount of money you spend on junk food and empty-calorie food and increasing the amount of money you spend on healthy food.

Second, you need to motivate yourself. Change is usually difficult for most people. Figure out what it will take for you to get motivated. Put pictures on your refrigerator. If you have supportive friends, tell them and have them give you their support. If your friends are negative naysayers, don't tell them. They will only drag you down. Picture yourself one year from now, five years from now. Strive toward that goal. Make the commitment.

Join local fitness groups. On weekends, go out with the local bicycle riding group. Seek out a Meet Up group that goes walking or hiking. Join a gym. Hire a personal trainer. Once you make the mental and financial commitment, you're more likely to see it through and not quit.

One of the most important things to focus on, if not the most important, is the calorie to nutrient ratio of the food you eat. Studies have shown that the less you eat, the longer you can live (I'm not speaking about starving, obviously.) I like to say that we are over-fed and under-nourished. Secondly is the importance of fasting, detoxing, and cleansing. And last but not least, the importance of exercise.

Detox and Fast

The first thing I suggest you do when you begin your new healthy lifestyle is to do a **detox** and **fast** to reset your system and give your internal organs a break. The best detox program I have used over the past 20 years is the Arise and Shine 28-Day Detox. I like their product so much, I became a distributor for them. If you want to order the kit, you can get it on my website. The cost is $250. Before you say, "I can't afford $250," keep in mind that you won't have to spend any money on groceries, so you will simply be transferring your grocery bill to your health bill. There are a couple other good detox/cleanse products I like put out by various nutraceutical companies including Metagenics, Douglas Labs, and Biotics.

I would also suggest doing a **juice fast**. You can do a juice fast before your detox/fast or as you're coming off your detox/fast. Or if you decided not to do the detox/fast at all, you can try starting with a 3-day juice fast, if that is more comfortable for you.

Probiotics to assist your intestinal flora and keep your gut healthy.

Enzymes to help your digestion and allow everything to work the way it's supposed to.

Meal Replacement

As you work back into a normal, healthy diet, one thing you can do is to include one meal replacement shake per day, in order to get your nutrients without all the calories. My favorite is Shakeology by Beach Body. Again, because I like it so much, I sell it on my website.

Vitamins

I'm a firm believer in vitamins. I find it interesting that there are doctors who come out and say that vitamins are either worthless or dangerous. I'm not sure how they can be dangerous to your health, if they are worthless and provide no value. Admittedly, there are good quality vitamins and bad quality vitamins. If you're paying under $20 for a 30-day supply of vitamins, I would question the quality. I've used Beach Body, Jay Robb, Biotics, Douglas Labs, and a few others. I'm sure there are other good brands out there. Check your local health food store. Read the labels!

Fresh Lemon Water. Lemons help to detox your liver, and it actually alkalizes your body. Remember, you don't want to be acidic. Most of us are way too acidic. (You can check your acid/alkaline numbers with pH strips.) "A glass of lemon juice contains less than 25 calories. It is a rich source of nutrients like calcium, potassium, vitamin C and pectin fiber. It also has medicinal values and antibacterial properties. It also contains traces of iron and vitamin A. Lemon, a fruit popular for its therapeutic properties, helps maintain your immune system and thus, protects you from the clutches of most types of infections. It also plays the role of a blood purifier. Lemon is a fabulous antiseptic and lime-water juice also works wonders for people having heart problems, owing to its high potassium content." (www.foodmatters.tv)

At a bare minimum, that's what you should start with. But that's just the beginning. Then, you have to cut out all the bad food and replace it with all the good food.

Food

Following is a list of things I suggest you keep in your kitchen and take every day:

Super-foods. See the list above. Add as many of these as possible to your diet. Load up your kitchen. You can juice them, cook with them, put them in your salad, etc. Work them into your diet.

You can buy Super-foods at places like Whole Foods, Sprouts, Mothers, etc.

Apple Cider Vinegar. I take one tablespoon per day, usually in the morning. Apple Cider Vinegar has a number of healthy benefits including:

- Wards off the flu
- Dissolves Kidney Stones
- Detoxifies the body

- Balances pH
- Relieves Heartburn
- Helps relieve nausea
- Relieves Allergies
- Lowers glucose levels
- Appetite suppressant
- Helps relieves migraines
- Helps relieve sinus pressure
- Lowers blood pressure
- Lowers cholesterol
- Kills or slows the growth of cancer cells
- Reduces inflammation
- Relieves arthritis

Flax Seed Oil – I suggest one tablespoon per day. This has the good fats that you need.

Flax seeds – These are great to put in a smoothie or sprinkle on your cereal or yogurt. Flax seeds will help keep your colon clean.

Chia seeds – These act as scrubbing bubbles that keep your colon clean. They are an excellent source of protein, essential fatty acids, and fiber.

Coconut Oil – Replace your other cooking oils with coconut oil to reduce stress, have healthier skin, hair and nails while also obtaining essential vitamins.

Coconut Milk – To regulate your digestive system, coconut milk can provide the soothing effects that you're after.

Coconut Water – By consuming coconut water on a daily basis, you're able to give your body the boost it needs.

Avocado – The Good Fat. It can be added on your salad or put on your burrito, to name a couple uses. It provides a full flavor, but also provides essential vitamins and nutrients.

Garlic – It has powerful antiviral, antiseptic and antibiotic properties. Garlic helps stimulate the liver into producing detoxification enzymes that help filter toxins from the digestive system.

Onions – Onions have anti-septic and anti-bacterial properties, plus they can taste good in almost any meal.

Ginger – Ginger is great for your digestive system.

Fermented Foods

- Kefir
- Yogurt
- Sauerkraut
- Kimchi

Chili Peppers – Chili peppers will raise your endorphin levels. They contain a lot of Vitamin C and beta-carotene. Being high in anti-oxidants, it's helpful for fighting colds, coughs, sinus issues, etc. Chili peppers also increase your metabolism which burns more calories.

Herbs and Spices

Cilantro – Can be considered both a spice and an herb. It is also known as coriander or Chinese parsley. It contains phytonutrients and antioxidants. It is a good source of Vitamins A, C, and K. Cilantro is great for detoxing the body of mercury, aluminum, lead, and cadmium.

Turmeric

- Anti-inflammatory
- Anti-biotic
- Antiseptic
- Analgesic
- Speeds up wound healing
- Improves digestion

- Blood purifier
- Skin tonic
- Improves asthma
- Anti-arthritic
- Prevents gas and bloating
- Lowers cholesterol
- Heals stomach ulcers
- Improves skin conditions
- Aids in fat metabolism and weight management

Cayenne Pepper

- Boosts metabolism
- Suppresses hunger
- Normalizes blood sugar

Supplements, Vitamins, Minerals

Iodine

- Forms thyroid hormone
- Eliminates heavy metals
- Lowers risk of diabetes
- Helps control weight
- Lowers blood pressure
- Assists in detoxification
- Protects from radiation

CoQ10 – This is good for your heart and cardiovascular system. If you are going to be working out, then you want to make sure your heart is healthy enough to withstand the strain. It lowers your resting heart rate and increases endurance. It has the ability to generate cellular energy and boost metabolism. It also helps to regulate the fats and sugars in your blood.

Stevia – Stevia is a natural sweetener that is finally gaining some popularity. Like other sweeteners, it has its own unique flavor, so you may have to get used to it. Too much could taste a little bitter, so you don't need a lot. Take a look in your local health food store, and see what brands they have. You can get it in powder or liquid form.

Hydrochloric Acid (HCl) – Key to digestion, HCl allows the enzyme pepsin to begin digestion in the stomach and kills microorganisms in food. HCl is also needed for mineral absorption including Calcium, iron, and zinc. Lack of HCl causes maldigestion and can lead to candida.

Green tea – High in antioxidants and polyphenol catechins, green tea is a great replacement for coffee or other beverages you normally drink throughout the day. Green tea with caffeine has been shown to reduce body weight, body mass index, and your waistline.

Protein Powder – There are many protein powders on the market today. I like Jay Robb's Egg White Protein. It's a bit expensive, but I know Jay makes a good product. Whey protein is probably the most popular, but some people are allergic to whey products. Nowadays there are protein powders made from alternative sources such as egg whites, peas, etc. You may want to try a different one each month until you find one that you like. They all have different tastes and consistencies, and they may affect your digestive system differently. If the protein powder you're taking upsets your stomach, try a different brand.

Some general lifestyle changes:

- Reduce the amount of calories you eat. Keep in mind the calorie to nutrient ratio.
- Set aside two hours once a week to eat whatever you want.
- Keep a positive attitude
- Become a student of wellness

- If you mess up, don't worry about it. Just regroup and start again
- When you eat, eat. Don't eat and walk. Don't eat and watch TV.
- Eat slowly. Enjoy your meal. Helps digestion.
- Take healthy snacks with you to work, so you don't get tempted by the vending machines
- Watch your portions
- Eat fruits and vegetables as snacks
- Drink water throughout the day. About a half ounce per pound of body weight.
- Drink a glass of water 30 minutes before a meal
- Exercise at least 30 minutes per day
- Get enough sleep
- Take time to relax – meditate, massage, beach, mountains, etc.

There are various ways to lose weight. We've discussed fasting, cleansing, detoxing, increasing your input of healthy whole foods, excluding or reducing bad foods, etc. We talked about vitamins and minerals, enzymes, probiotics, and digestion. Another weight loss plan we didn't really discuss is thermogenics. This is a form of heating up your body and increasing your metabolism. This can be accomplished in a number of ways. Since your thyroid controls your metabolism, you can focus on boosting your thyroid by taking iodine, herbal supplements, or certain super-foods. You can also cause thermogenics through products that use chemical stimulants such as HydroxyCut. This will burn calories, but it's not in the realm of natural remedies. Another way is through hormone replacement therapy which I won't cover in this book.

Conclusion

Once again, I want to thank you for purchasing this book. I hope it gives you the knowledge and motivation to get started on your new healthy life! Don't put it off. I hope and pray you don't just read this, set it to the side, and decide to do nothing.

I read that one quarter of all men and one half of all women are dieting to lose weight. Here's the catch. Losing the weight is not always the hard part. You can lose weight doing any number of fad diets. Keeping the weight off is the hard part. It is estimated that 75%-90% of all people who lose weight gain it all back within one to three years. The key, as I hope you've gotten from reading this book, is in leading a healthy lifestyle and not doing a diet.

One thing that pains me is when people come to me with health issues, explaining how they are in pain, are overweight, have diabetes, high blood pressure, high cholesterol, etc., and then make the conscious decision not to do anything about it – even after I've told them how they can get healthy. Don't be one of those people. You can be healthy. You can lose weight. You can reduce your risk of disease. You don't have to take a dozen pharmaceutical drugs every day. So, if you're ready to be healthy, then make the commitment to start today.

If you go to my website, you can sign up for a Wellness Assessment. I will send you a questionnaire, and once you fill it out, I will put together a report that will tell you where your health is lacking and what you need.

www.ulti-health.com and www.billystixworkout.com

10 Amazing Vegan Recipes

The vegan diet eliminates all animal products and is a step up from a vegetarian diet in regards to dietary restrictions. The recipes in this book only use vegetables, grains, nuts, legumes, seeds and fruits and avoid the use of any animal product including dairy products, gelatin or anything else produced from animals.

Vegans need to supplement the lack of protein from animal sources in their diet with legumes, tofu, wheat bread, kale, tofu and other non-animal foods that are high in protein. The vegan diet offers a high level of protection against cardiovascular disease, diabetes, heart problems and other chronic illnesses with the positive health benefits that fruits and vegetables provide. Included in this guide are 10 great vegan recipes that are delicious and easy to make.

Vegan Black Bean Soup

This black bean soup is easy to make and offers a great source of protein. It has a nice zesty flavor and includes tomatoes, corn, onion, garlic and spices for a healthy and satisfying combination.

Ingredients:

- 1 tablespoon olive oil
- 3 carrots, chopped
- 2 tablespoons chili powder
- 1 can crushed tomatoes, 14.5 ounce
- 4 cans of black beans, 15 ounce
- 1 teaspoon black pepper
- 1 tablespoon ground cumin
- 4 cups vegetable broth
- 1 can whole kernel corn, 15 ounce
- 3 cloves garlic, chopped
- 1 celery stalk, chopped
- 1 large onion, chopped
- 1 teaspoon cumin

Directions:

1. Heat oil on medium heat in large pot.

2. Sauté carrots, garlic, celery and onion for 4 to 5 minutes.

3. Add cumin, black pepper and chili powder and cook for 1 minute.

4. Add vegetable broth, corn and 2 cans of beans.

5. Blend 2 other cans of black beans and tomatoes until smooth.

6. Stir into soup and reduce heat to simmer for 15-18 minutes.

Tip: You can use frozen corn in this recipe if you prefer.

Calories: This recipe serves 8 at 417 calories per serving.

Vegan Garbanzo Stir Fry

This is a filling and satisfying stir fry for a vegan diet that allows you to add extra ingredients and vegetables as you see fit. It works great as it is or you can customize it as you see fit with your own veggies.

Ingredients:

- 1 can garbanzo beans, 15 ounce, drained and rinsed
- 1 large zucchini sliced and halved
- 2 tablespoons extra virgin olive oil
- 1 tablespoon fresh cilantro, chopped
- 1 tablespoon fresh basil, chopped
- 1 teaspoon fresh ground black pepper
- 1 tomato, seeded and chopped
- ½ cup mushrooms, sliced
- 1 tablespoon chopped fresh oregano
- 2 cloves garlic, minced

Directions:

1. Heat oil on medium heat in a large skillet.

2. Add zucchini and garbanzo beans.

3. Add garlic and pepper and stir well.

4. Cook for 10 minutes, covered and stir occasionally.

5. Add mushrooms and cilantro and stir occasionally.

6. Add fresh herbs and stir.

7. Put chopped tomato on top and cover and let steam for 2-3 minutes.

8. Serve right away.

Tip: You can adjust this recipe by adding different vegetables such as sugar snap peas, corn and carrots.

Calories: This recipe serves 2 at 432 calories per serving.

Vegan Quinoa Tabouli

This changes up traditional tabouli by using Quinoa, a healthy grain. It tastes just as good as bulgur if not better, and it is a great side dish that can be refrigerated for a while.

Ingredients:

- 3 tomatoes, seeded and diced
- 1 cup fresh parsley, chopped
- ¼ cup lemon juice
- ½ teaspoon salt
- ¼ cup olive oil
- 2 carrots, grated
- 2 cups water
- 1 cup of Quinoa
- 1 cucumber diced
- 3 green onions, diced

Directions:

1. Rinse Quinoa under cold water.

2. Bring 2 cups of water to boil.

3. Add Quinoa and a small pinch of sea salt.

4. Reduce heat and simmer 14 minutes.

5. Cool to room temperature and use a fork to fluff.

6. Combine remainder of ingredients and mix.

7. Stir in Quinoa and cool in refrigerator before serving.

Tip: Be sure to wash the Quinoa to remove any residue before boiling it.

Calories: This recipe serves 4 at 305 calories per serving.

Vegan Quinoa and Black Beans

This is a flavorful and healthy alternative to black beans and rice, as Quinoa is higher in protein. It is a quick and easy satisfying dish that looks great once done and is very healthy.

Ingredients:

- 1 onion, chopped
- 1 teaspoon extra virgin olive oil
- ½ teaspoon fresh ground black pepper.
- ½ teaspoon cayenne pepper
- 1 cup corn kernels, frozen
- 1 cup Quinoa
- 3 cloves garlic, chopped
- 1 teaspoon ground cumin
- 1 ½ cups vegetable broth
- 2 cans black beans, 15 ounce, drained and rinsed
- ½ cup fresh cilantro, chopped
- Salt to taste

Directions:

1. Heat oil in saucepan on medium heat.

2. Saute garlic and onion about 10 minutes until browned.

3. Add Quinoa to mixture and add vegetable broth.

4. Add cumin, salt, black pepper and cayenne pepper.

5. Bring to a boil.

6. Reduce heat, cover and simmer until Quinoa is tender.

7. Add frozen corn and simmer 5 minutes.

8. Add cilantro and black beans.

Tip: You can add zucchini, tomatoes and other cooked vegetables to this dish at the last step.

Calories: This recipe serves 4 at 511 calories per serving.

Lentils and Spinach

This recipe is based on the standard Indian daal (lentil) recipe and turns out nicely. It can be served with a potato or with rice and works great with other vegetable entrees or side dishes.

Ingredients:

- 1 package frozen spinach, 10 ounces
- 2 cups water
- 3 cloves garlic, crushed
- ½ cup lentils
- 2 cloves garlic, minced
- 1 teaspoon ground black pepper
- 1 teaspoon sea salt
- 2 white onions sliced into ½ rings
- 1 teaspoon ground cumin
- 1 tablespoon extra-virgin olive oil

Directions:

1. Heat oil in a large saucepan on medium heat.

2. Sautee onion for 10 minutes until golden in color.

3. Add minced garlic and sauté for 1-2 minutes.

4. Add lentils and water to saucepan and bring to boil.

5. Cover and simmer for 30 to 35 minutes.

6. Cook the spinach in the microwave based on directions.

7. Add cumin, salt, pepper, crushed garlic and spinach to lentils.

8. Cover and simmer 10 minutes.

Tip: You can substitute fresh spinach for frozen in this recipe.

Calories: This recipe serves 2 at 327 calories per serving.

Vegan Potato Curry

This is a filling and delicious potato curry with several spices and rich ingredients. It can be eaten as both a main dish and a side dish and it goes nicely with many other vegan recipes.

Ingredients:

- 4 russet potatoes, peeled and cubed
- 1 large onion, diced
- 1 can of coconut milk, 14 ounce
- 1 can of peas, 15 ounce, drained
- 1 tablespoon fresh ginger, minced
- 1 can garbanzo beans, 15 ounce, rinsed and drained
- 1 can diced tomatoes, 15 ounce
- 4 cloves garlic, minced
- 2 teaspoons ground cumin
- 1 ½ teaspoons cayenne pepper
- 4 teaspoons curry powder
- 4 teaspoons garam masala
- 2 tablespoons vegetable oil

Directions:

1. Put potatoes in a large saucepan and add enough water to cover, and a pinch of sea salt.

2. Bring to a boil on high, reduce to simmer for 15 minutes.

3. Drain and allow to steam dry.

4. Heat vegetable oil on medium heat in a large skillet.

5. Add garlic and onion and sauté until onion is softened, about 6-8 minutes.

6. Add spices, ginger and salt and cook for 3 minutes.

7. Add peas, garbanzo beans, tomatoes and potatoes.

8. Add coconut milk and heat to simmer for 8 to 10 minutes.

Tip: Goes well with basmati rice or Indian naan.

Calories: This recipe serves 8 at 483 calories per serving.

Vegan Cuban Beans and Rice

This is based on authentic Cuban beans and rice and goes great in a tortilla or as a side dish. It is very filling and is very easy to prepare, and it can be stored and eaten later after making it.

Ingredients:

- 1 cup white rice, uncooked
- 1 large green bell pepper, chopped
- 1 large onion, chopped
- 4 tablespoons tomato paste
- 1 teaspoon sea salt
- 1 can kidney beans, drained (reserve the liquid)
- 1 tablespoon extra-virgin olive oil
- 3 garlic cloves, minced

Directions:

1. Heat oil on medium heat in saucepan.
2. Add garlic, bell pepper and onion. Sautee for 10 minutes.
3. Add tomato paste and sea salt and cook on low for 3 minutes.
4. Add beans and rice.
5. Add liquid from beans into a measuring cup and add water to increase it to 2 ½ cups.
6. Add liquid to beans and rice and cook for 45 to 50 minutes or until liquid is absorbed.

Tip: Allow this to sit overnight for a richer flavor the next day.

Calories: This recipe serves 6 at 402 calories per serving.

Vegan Ginger Garlic Tofu

Tofu is a staple food for any vegan diet, as it is rich in protein and has many health benefits. This is an easy to make ginger garlic tofu recipe that can be stored and eaten later or right away.

Ingredients:

- 3 tablespoons sesame oil
- 2 pounds firm tofu
- 2 teaspoons ginger, minced
- 2 teaspoons garlic, minced
- 1 tablespoon tamari

Directions:

1. Heat oil on medium heat in a skillet.
2. Add garlic and ginger and cook for 2 minutes.
3. Add tamari and tofu and stir.
4. Cover and cook for 25 to 30 minutes.

Tip: This tofu goes great with rice and steamed vegetables.

Calories: This recipe serves 4 at 257 calories per serving.

Vegan Aloo Matar

Aloo matar is an Indian potato dish in a tomato puree that is easy to make and goes great with fresh Indian naan or Basmati rice. It's also a great option for a side dish.

Ingredients:

- ½ cup tomato puree
- 2 ½ tablespoons garam masala
- ¼ cup vegetable oil
- 3 potatoes, peeled and cubed
- 2 medium onions, chopped
- 1 tablespoon ginger, minced
- 1 tablespoon garlic, minced
- 1 bay leaf
- 1 teaspoon brown sugar
- 2 tablespoons fresh cilantro, chopped
- 2 teaspoons paprika
- 1 cup frozen peas

Directions:

1. Heat oil on a skillet on medium.

2. Add ginger, garlic, onions and bay leaf.

3. Cook until onions are golden brown.

4. Add potatoes and peas and cover and cook for 15 minutes.

5. Remove bay leaf.

6. Add the rest of the ingredients except the cilantro and cook for 10 minutes.

7. Add cilantro and cook for 2 minutes.

Tip: You can precook the potatoes with sea salt and pepper to speed the cooking time up.

Calories: This recipe serves 4 at 312 calories per serving.

Vegan Avocado Tacos

These tacos are fast and easy and use healthy avocado. They are addictive and they go well with vegan Mexican entrees and other types of vegan cuisine or they are great just as a snack.

Ingredients:

- 3 avocados, peeled and mashed
- 1/2 small onion, diced
- ¼ teaspoon sea salt
- ¼ teaspoon garlic powder
- 1 jalapeno pepper, seeded and chopped
- 2 tablespoons cilantro leaves, chopped
- 12 corn tortillas

Directions:

1. Preheat oven to 325 F.
2. Add garlic powder, sea salt, peppers, onions and avocados in a bowl and mix.
3. Arrange corn tortillas on a baking sheet and heat in oven for 2-4 minutes.
4. Spread avocado mixture on tortillas and garnish with cilantro.

Tip: If you prefer it to be mild take the jalapeno out of the recipe.

Calories: This recipe serves 6 at 313 calories per serving.

10 Amazing Paleo Recipes

The Paleo diet attempts to create the diet that Paleolithic humans ate prior to the advent of modern agriculture, and is based on the idea that a modern diet has resulted in obesity and other health problems. The Paleo diet has grown in popularity in recent times because it can reduce a person's risk of chronic illnesses and improve overall health.

The diet allows you to eat only what a caveman would eat, and the creators of the Paleo diet suggest that many of the modern chronic illnesses and health problems that we experience are the result of a grain based diet. A modern diet results in a higher predisposition to Type II diabetes, high blood pressure, and other health problems. Below are ten great Paleo diet recipes to try out that include delicious whole foods and will help you stick to the diet's guidelines.

Paleo Caribbean Jerk Chicken

This jerk chicken recipe is spicy and healthy, and it includes several delicious spices. It can be eaten right after cooking or it can be stored in the fridge for a few days, and it goes well with salad or a veggie side dish.

Ingredients:

- 1 ½ pounds chicken thighs or breasts, boneless and skinless
- 1 tablespoon extra-virgin olive oil
- 3 tablespoons extra-virgin olive oil
- 1 ½ teaspoon ground black pepper
- 1 teaspoon red paprika
- ½ teaspoon garlic powder
- 1 teaspoon thyme
- ½ teaspoon cayenne pepper
- 1 teaspoon cumin
- ½ teaspoon sea salt

Directions:

1. Preheat oven to 375 F.

2. Cut chicken into approximately 1 inch pieces.

3. Mix together spices in a bowl.

4. Add spices to the chicken including 1 tablespoon extra-virgin olive oil.

5. Add 3 tablespoons of oil in a non-stick frying pan. When the oil is hot, add the chicken pieces.

6. Stir fry the chicken until it is browned.

7. Put chicken in a baking dish and cover.

8. Bake for 7 to 9 minutes.

9. Remove chicken from oven and serve.

Tip: You can store this chicken in the fridge after you make it as it reheats nicely.

Calories: This recipe serves 4 at 451.25 calories per serving.

Paleo Salmon

This is an easy recipe for salmon that is delicious and a great source of healthy protein on the Paleo diet. Every ingredient is approved for the diet and it takes only minutes to prepare.

Ingredients:

- 1 tablespoon fresh lemon juice
- 4 tablespoons extra virgin olive oil
- 1 tablespoon fresh parsley
- A pinch of dill weed
- 1 teaspoon ground black pepper
- 3 garlic cloves, minced
- 1 teaspoon sea salt
- 2 salmon fillet, 6 oz.

Directions:

1. Mix ingredients except for salmon in a mixing bowl.

2. Put salmon fillets in a baking dish and cover with marinade.

3. Marinate for 1 hour, turn salmon at least once.

4. Cover salmon in aluminum foil and pour marinade inside.

5. Seal and place fillets in baking dish.

6. Bake for 40 to 45 minutes until salmon.

Tip: You can add more garlic to make it even healthier (if you love garlic that is).

Calories: This recipe serves 2 at 488 calories per serving.

Garlic Mashed Cauliflower

On the Paleo diet cauliflower works as a potato replacement and this recipe is a delicious and healthy cauliflower mashed potato that goes well as a side dish for any Paleo protein recipe.

Ingredients:

- 1 head of cauliflower, chopped roughly
- 3 cloves of garlic, chopped
- 1 teaspoon of sea salt
- 2 tablespoons of butter (grass fed)
- 1 teaspoon fresh ground black pepper

Directions:

1. Fill up a large stock pot with 2 inches of water.

2. Set the stove on high and put a steamer insert in the pot and cover.

3. Steam cauliflower and garlic for approximately 10 minutes.

4. Drain garlic and cauliflower in colander.

5. Put garlic, cauliflower, butter, sea salt and pepper into food processor.

6. Process until mixture is a smooth puree.

Tip: You can use garlic powder if you don't have fresh garlic on hand and you can substitute a different fat for butter such as lard or olive oil.

Calories: This recipe serves 2 at 144 calories per serving.

Paleo Grilled Zucchini

Grilled zucchini is an amazing Paleo veggie side dish that goes great with several of the protein entrees and zucchini has several health benefits. This is a simple grilled zucchini that is flavorful and easy to make.

Ingredients:

- 2 zucchinis, cut lengthwise
- 1 tablespoon extra-virgin olive oil
- 1 teaspoon sea salt
- ½ teaspoon black pepper
- ½ teaspoon garlic powder
- 1 teaspoon Italian seasoning
- 2 tablespoons balsamic vinegar

Directions:

1. Put grill on medium low heat.

2. Brush zucchini with olive oil.

3. Sprinkle sea salt, pepper, garlic powder and Italian seasoning on zucchini.

4. Brush balsamic vinegar on zucchini.

5. Cook for 4 to 5 minutes each side.

Tip: You can marinade the zucchini for an hour to make it more flavorful.

Calories: This recipe serves 2 at 102 calories per serving.

Paleo Guacamole

Guacamole is a healthy Paleo side that can be eaten with romaine lettuce wraps, used as a condiment for burgers and sandwiches, and has many other uses. This guacamole only takes minutes to make.

Ingredients:

- 3 ripe avocados, peeled
- A pinch of sea salt and pepper
- 1 tablespoon chopped cilantro
- 1 jalapeno pepper, seeded and diced
- 2 cloves garlic, minced
- 1 ½ Roma tomatoes, diced
- 1 ½ small onion, minced
- Juice of 1 lime

Directions:

1. Smash avocados in a bowl with a fork thoroughly and add lime juice.

2. Add rest of ingredients and use fork to mix.

Tip: You can use red onion in this recipe or other types of tomatoes.

Calories: This recipe serves 6 at 220 calories per serving.

Paleo Beef and Broccoli

This recipe combines two healthy Paleo foods, beef and broccoli, with delicious cashews and spices. It is easy to make and is a great choice for lunch or dinner, and takes approximately 45 minutes to fully cook.

Ingredients:

- 3 tablespoons honey
- 3 garlic cloves, minced
- 3 cups fresh broccoli florets
- ½ teaspoon sea salt
- 1 teaspoon pepper
- 1 cup gluten free soy sauce
- ½ cup toasted cashews
- 2 tablespoons coconut oil
- 1 pound flank steak, sliced thinly
- 1 teaspoon red pepper flakes
- 1 teaspoon fresh ginger, grated

Directions:

1. Whisk honey, soy sauce, garlic, red pepper flakes, ginger, and sea salt and pepper together.

2. Put sliced steak into a bowl and pour mixture on top.

3. Marinate in fridge for 1 hour.

4. Put a large pan on medium heat.

5. Add 1 tablespoon of coconut oil and add broccoli.

6. Cook broccoli until desired doneness and remove from pan.

7. Add 1 tablespoon of coconut oil and add meat/marinade.

8. Cook meat for 15 to 20 minutes or until no pink remains.

9. Add broccoli and cashews back into pan and cook for 2 more minutes.

Tip: You can steam the broccoli separately and add it back in at the last step if you have a steamer.

Calories: This recipe serves 4 at 455 calories per serving.

Paleo Chicken Soup

Chicken soup goes great with many Paleo recipes and it is a healthy option for the diet. This chicken soup is very easy to make and has several great Paleo ingredients including fresh chicken, carrots, onion and more.

Ingredients:

- 1/4 teaspoon celery salt
- ½ teaspoon black pepper
- 1 skinless, boneless chicken breast, halved
- 1 onion, chopped
- 1 clove garlic, minced
- 2 cans chicken broth

Directions:

1. Bring chicken broth to boil on medium heat.

2. Add onion, garlic, carrots, pepper and celery salt.

3. Reduce heat to low

4. Add chicken breast and simmer for 20 minutes, covered.

5. Remove chicken breast and trim into chunks and return to pot.

Tip: You can add more vegetables like celery to this soup.

Calories: This recipe serves 2 at 263 calories per serving.

Paleo Broiled Chicken Breasts

This is a very easy way to make chicken using olive oil. The chicken turns out juicy and crisp on the outside, and it serves as a basic Paleo protein entree that you can add many different sides to.

Ingredients:

- 4 chicken breasts, bone in with skin
- 3 tablespoons extra virgin olive oil
- 2 teaspoons sea salt
- 1 teaspoon fresh ground black pepper
- 1 teaspoon fresh rosemary

Directions:

1. Preheat broiler on high and set 6 inches from heat source.

2. Rub olive oil on chicken breast and season with rosemary, salt and pepper.

3. Put the chicken skin side down in broiling pan.

4. Broil for 10-12 minutes on each side, or until chicken is fully cooked and thermometer reads at 165 F.

Tip: Add ¼ cup of water to broiling pan to use chicken juices as a baste for the chicken.

Calories: This recipe serves 4 at 375 calories per serving.

Paleo Sweet Potato Hash and Eggs

This is a hearty and delicious breakfast for the Paleo diet that includes sweet potatoes and eggs. It is relatively easy to make and if you have a food processor it will speed up the preparation.

Ingredients:

- 2 large sweet potatoes
- 1 teaspoon sea salt
- 1 teaspoon freshly ground black pepper
- 1 teaspoon garlic powder
- 1 teaspoon Italian seasoning
- 1 teaspoon onion powder
- 4 tablespoons butter (grass fed)
- 8 large eggs
- Salt and pepper for the eggs to taste

Directions:

1. Peel the sweet potatoes and cut them to fit in your food processor lengthwise.

2. Use the julienne blade on the food processor to shred the sweet potatoes or grate them by hand.

3. Put shredded sweet potato in a bowl and add onion and garlic powder, sea salt and pepper, and Italian seasoning.

4. Add butter to large cast iron skillet and turn on medium heat.

5. Add sweet potatoes to pan and stir fry for 2 minutes.

6. Cover and let cook for 5-6 more minutes until sweet potatoes are tender. Remove from pan.

7. Melt 1 tablespoon of butter in pan.

8. Add 2 eggs in pan.

9. Cover and cook for 3-4 minutes sunny side up or based on preferences for yolk runniness.

10. Slide out of pan onto top of hash, and repeat for steps 8-10 for the next 6 eggs.

Tip: You can use real onion and garlic as a replacement for the powders in this recipe. Reduce ingredients by half if you need to serve 2 people.

Calories: This recipe serves 4 at 306 calories per serving

Paleo Spinach Omelette

This Paleo omelette is easy to make and turns out nicely with fresh spinach. It is a low carb meal to start the day on or a great pre-workout meal, and it takes just minutes to prepare.

Ingredients:

- 4 eggs
- 2 cups baby spinach leaves, torn
- ½ teaspoon onion powder
- ½ teaspoon garlic powder
- 1 tablespoon olive oil
- Salt and pepper to taste

Directions:

1. Beat eggs in a large bowl.

2. Add baby spinach and Parmesan cheese.

3. Add salt, pepper, onion and garlic powder

4. Coat a large non-stick skillet with olive oil and add egg mixture and cook for 4-5 minutes, until it starts to set.

5. Flip with a spatula and cook for another 4-5 minutes.

6. Reduce heat and cook until desired level of doneness.

Tip: You can also add tomatoes, peppers and other ingredients in the second step as desired.

Calories: This recipe serves 2 at 197 calories per serving.

10 Amazing Gluten Free Recipes

Gluten free diets avoid any foods that have gluten, a protein found in wheat, rye, and barely. Gluten free diets are used to treat allergies to gluten and they are the only known treatment for certain illnesses like celiac disease. However, gluten sensitivity is also a common health problem that a gluten free diet can help with. It is thought that up to 10 percent of the population has sensitivity to gluten and may benefit from a gluten free diet.

The recipes in this book are carefully selected to be gluten free, and they are delicious meal choices. There are an infinite number of recipes that can exclude gluten, there can be numerous health benefits to these recipes. Cutting gluten out of your diet can help your body, and foods that need to be avoided include pasta, beer, breads, candies, cakes, cereals, cookies, many types of sauces, and other foods unless they are specifically labeled gluten free. The recipes in this book do not use any ingredients with gluten in them and are good choices for those with gluten sensitivities or who prefer to avoid gluten in general in their diet.

Gluten Free Stuffed Peppers

This stuffed pepper recipe is gluten free and easy to make. It uses rice, however rice is gluten free (except for prepared rice mixes). Do not purchase prepared rice mixes, instead just buy uncooked rice for this and other gluten free recipes that use rice.

Ingredients:

- 1 cup water
- 1 teaspoon Italian seasoning
- 2 cans tomato sauce, 8 ounces
- ½ teaspoon garlic powder
- ½ teaspoon onion powder
- Salt and pepper to taste
- 6 green bell peppers, whole
- 1 tablespoon Worcestershire sauce
- ½ cup uncooked brown or white rice
- 1 pound ground beef

Directions:

1. Preheat oven to 350 F.

2. Put rice in a saucepan and add water and increase heat to boil. Reduce heat, cover and cook for 20 minutes.

3. Cook beef in medium skillet until browned.

4. Remove tops and seeds of green peppers.

5. Put peppers on a baking dish with open sides facing up.

6. Mix rice, browned beef, 1 can of tomato sauce, and the rest of the ingredients.

7. Add the mixture into each pepper in an equal amount.

8. Pour second can of tomato sauce over peppers.

9. Bake for 1 hour and baste with sauce every 15 minutes.

Tip: Add mozzarella cheese or cheddar cheese at the last 5 minutes if preferred.

Calories: This recipe serves 4 at 360 calories per serving.

Gluten Free Garlic Mashed Potatoes

These mashed potatoes are healthy and easy to make, and offer a great alternative to wheat side dishes. They are gluten free and have a nice garlic flavor, and they are perfect with several dishes.

Ingredients:

- ¼ cup extra virgin olive oil
- 7 garlic cloves, peeled
- 2 tablespoons butter
- ¼ cup Parmesan cheese
- 6 potatoes, cubed and peeled
- ½ cup milk
- ½ teaspoon sea salt
- ¼ teaspoon black pepper

Directions:

1. Preheat oven to 350 F.

2. Put garlic cloves in baking dish. Add olive oil and bake for 20-25 minutes or until cloves are brown.

3. Add water to a large pot and bring to boil.

4. Add cubed potatoes and a pinch of sea salt and cook until tender.

5. Drain and transfer to large mixing bowl.

6. Add all of the rest of the ingredients to the bowl including garlic.

7. Use a masher or electric mixer to beat potatoes.

Tip: Add more Parmesan cheese for more flavor, you can be liberal with it in this recipe.

Calories: This recipe serves 6 at 284 calories per serving.

Gluten Free Quinoa

Quinoa is a grain that does not have gluten in it, and it is a great grain replacement for people who are on a gluten free diet. This is a nice Quinoa side dish that can go with any gluten free main.

Ingredients:

- 1 cup Quinoa, uncooked
- ¼ teaspoon sea salt
- 1 small onion, chopped
- 2 cloves of garlic, chopped
- 2 tablespoons parsley, chopped
- 1 tablespoon butter
- ½ tablespoon thyme, chopped
- 2 cups vegetable broth

Directions:

1. Melt butter in a large saucepan on medium heat.

2. Add Quinoa and brown for 5 minutes.

3. Add broth and increase heat to boiling.

4. Reduce heat and simmer for 14 minutes.

5. Add Quinoa to bowl with the rest of the ingredients and toss together.

Tip: Sprinkle some fresh lemon juice at the end if desired.

Calories: This recipe serves 4 at 201 calories per serving.

Gluten Free Artichoke Spinach Dip

This is a very rich but delicious artichoke spinach dip, and it does not have any gluten in it. It can be used with gluten free chips or as a vegetable dip, and it can be made quickly.

Ingredients:

- 1 can artichoke hearts, 14 ounce, drained
- ½ tablespoon garlic, minced
- 1 cup shredded mozzarella cheese
- ½ cup sour cream
- ½ cup heavy cream
- ¼ cup Parmesan cheese
- ¼ cup grated Romano cheese
- 1 package frozen chopped spinach, 10 ounce

Directions:

1. Preheat oven to 350 F.

2. Add artichoke hearts, Parmesan and Romano cheese, and garlic to a blender or food processor and pulse until chopped.

3. Add sour and heavy cream, spinach and mozzarella cheese in a medium bowl.

4. Add artichoke mixture to bowl.

5. Add spinach and artichoke mixture to a greased 9x13 baking dish.

6. Bake for 25 minutes or until cheese melts.

Tip: Try adding Asiago cheese in the mix to make the dip sharper in flavor.

Calories: This recipe serves 4 at 313 calories per serving.

Gluten Free Chicken Salad

This chicken salad recipe takes just minutes to make and is completely gluten free. This is an addictive chicken salad that can be served warm or cold, and it can be eaten with gluten free chips, in lettuce wraps, or with gluten free bread.

Ingredients:

- 2 celery stalks, chopped
- 2 dill pickles, chopped
- ½ red onion, diced
- 3 tablespoons mayonnaise
- 1 cooked boneless chicken breast, chopped
- ¼ teaspoon garlic powder
- ¼ teaspoon sea salt
- ¼ teaspoon pepper

Directions:

1. Combine chopped chicken with all ingredients.

2. Serve immediately or refrigerate.

Tip: If you prefer sweet pickles you can use sweet pickle relish instead of dill pickles.

Calories: This recipe serves 2 at 251 calories per serving.

Gluten Free Black Beans and Rice

This is a quick recipe for black beans and rice, and it is a great side dish. It goes well with salsa and you can adjust the spices in the recipe based on your preferences.

Ingredients:

- 1 large onion, chopped
- 2 cloves garlic, minced
- 1 can black beans, 15 ounce, undrained
- 1 can stewed tomatoes, 15 ounce
- 1 tablespoon fresh oregano, chopped
- ½ teaspoon garlic powder
- 1 tablespoon olive oil
- 1 ½ cups instant brown rice, uncooked

Directions:

1. Heat oil on medium high heat.

2. Add onion and garlic, cook until onion is tender.

3. And tomatoes, beans, garlic powder and oregano.

4. Increase heat to boiling and stir in rice.

5. Cover and simmer for 10 minutes or until rice absorbs liquid.

Tip: Add cumin and chili powder if you want to give it more of a chili flavor.

Calories: This recipe serves 4 at 454 calories per serving.

Gluten Free Blackened Chicken

This blackened chicken recipe is perfect for a summer meal and goes great with barbecue foods or with fresh vegetable sides and mashed potatoes. It is gluten free and takes minutes to prepare.

Ingredients:

- 2 chicken breasts, skinless and boneless
- ¼ teaspoon onion powder
- ¼ teaspoon ground black pepper
- ¼ teaspoon dried thyme
- ¼ teaspoon ground cumin
- ½ teaspoon red paprika
- 1/8 teaspoon sea salt
- ¼ teaspoon cayenne pepper
- 1 tablespoon olive oil or cooking spray

Directions:

1. Preheat oven to 350 F.
2. Heat a cast iron skillet until smoking hot.
3. Add spices together in a small mixing bowl.
4. Oil the chicken breasts with olive oil or cooking spray on both sides.
5. Coat the chicken breasts with the spice mix.
6. Put the chicken on the hot skillet and cook for 1 minute on each side.
7. Put chicken breasts on a lightly greased baking pan.
8. Bake about 8 minutes or until the chicken is not pink in the middle.

Tip: Turn your vent on as this recipe can create a lot of smoke.

Calories: This recipe serves 2 at 283 calories per serving.

Gluten Free Sirloin Steak

There's nothing quite like a great steak, and this recipe is gluten free and very easy to make as long as you have a grill ready to go. This steak uses butter and garlic for flavoring and it can be ready in less than 30 minutes.

Ingredients:

- 4 pounds sirloin steak
- 6 garlic cloves, minced
- 1/3 cup butter
- 2 teaspoons garlic powder
- Salt and pepper to taste

Directions:

1. Preheat grill on high.

2. Melt butter in saucepan on low heat and add garlic and garlic powder.

3. Season steaks with salt and pepper and brush with butter.

4. Grill 5 minutes each side or until preferred doneness. Brush with garlic butter while grilling.

Tip: You can avoid the garlic powder if you prefer a less powerful garlic flavor.

Calories: This recipe serves 8 at 495 calories per serving.

Gluten Free Cabbage Rolls

These cabbage rolls are completely gluten free and are tender and delicious as they are slow cooked to perfection. They have a nice tomato sauce and the preparation is relatively easy.

Ingredients:

- 12 cabbage leaves
- 1 teaspoon sea salt
- 1 teaspoon ground black pepper
- 1 can of tomato sauce, 8 ounce
- ¼ cup milk
- 1 large onion, minced
- 1 tablespoon Worcestershire sauce
- 1 tablespoon brown sugar
- 1 pound ground beef
- 1 tablespoon lemon juice
- 1 egg, beaten
- 1 cup white rice, cooked
- ½ teaspoon paprika

Directions:

1. Add water to a large pot and bring to boil. Add cabbage leaves and boil for 2 minutes and drain.

2. Add cooked rice, beef, onion, egg, milk, salt and pepper in a large mixing bowl and mix thoroughly.

3. Put about a quarter cup of the meat mixture into each cabbage leaf.

4. Roll up the leaves and tuck in the ends.

5. Mix Worcestershire sauce, tomato sauce, brown sugar and lemon juice and pour over cabbage rolls.

6. Put rolls in slow cooker and cook for 8 hours on low.

Tip: You can also freeze the cabbage head and thaw it to make the leaves wilt and avoid having to boil them.

Calories: This recipe serves 4 at 445 calories per serving.

Gluten Free Mushroom Risotto

This mushroom risotto is very healthy and can be served as a side dish or even a main course. It is gluten free and works as a great side dish to steak, chicken or fish entrees.

Ingredients:

- 1 cup milk (soy milk, coconut milk, almond milk)
- 1 tablespoon extra-virgin olive oil
- 2 medium onions, chopped finely
- 1 tablespoon parsley, minced
- 1 ½ cup mushrooms, sliced
- ¼ cup heavy cream
- 1 cup Arborio rice, uncooked
- 1 tablespoon butter
- ½ teaspoon sea salt
- ½ teaspoon pepper
- 1 cup Parmesan cheese, grated
- 2 cloves garlic, minced

Directions:

1. Heat oil on medium high in a large skillet.

2. Sautee garlic and onion until onion is slightly brown.

3. Add parsley salt and pepper and cook for 1-2 minutes.

4. Add mushrooms and reduce heat to low.

5. Cook mushrooms until softened.

6. And rice, milk and cream and heat until simmering.

7. Add vegetable stock to rice one cup at a time. Add the next cup once the first is fully absorbed.

8. Add butter and Parmesan cheese once the final cup of vegetable stock has been added.

Tip: Be sure to use Arborio rice with this recipe to ensure that it turns out with the right consistency.

Calories: This recipe serves 6 at 332 calories per serving.

Appendix A – Fitness Goals: Let's Begin

What are your fitness goals?

_____

_____

_____

_____

(ie. Lose 20 lbs, get more flexibility, gain strength, etc)

What is your current weight? _____

What is your goal weight? _____

What are your measurements?

      Chest _____

      Waist _____

      Hips _____

      Neck _____

      Biceps _____

      Thighs _____

      Calves _____

What is your body fat percentage? _____

What is your resting heart rate? _____ bpm (beats/min)

How long has it been since you've exercised regularly?

_____

Do you have a time frame?

_____

(ie. Need to lose 10lbs in 3 months for a wedding, etc.)

Write down everything you eat and drink for three days.

Answer these questions every month for six months.

Take a picture of yourself. Write the date on it. Put in on your refrigerator or your mirror. (You may not notice the change in your body, so you need a reference.)

Appendix B – Health Suggestions from Other Professionals

Felicia Drury Kliment

Nearly raw potatoes

Ice pack on the lower abdomen to take away the appetite

Raw honey. Contains amylase which help digestion

Raw milk and butter. Contains lipase and protease which breaks down fat and protein

Raw beefsteak

Avocados and bananas

Vitamin E to normalize thyroid function and neutralizes the poisonous by-products of saturated oils.

ChitoPlex

Coconut and Flaxseed oil

Raw carrots

Acidic, sour-tasting foods such as grape juice, vinegar, and yogurt

Eating several small meals

Blackstrap-lemon drink to detox the liver

Ice water before a meal

(I don't agree with everything on her list, but that just shows how there are many different opinions on what is healthy.)

Elson M. Haas

1. Consume less (bad) fat

2. Consume less red meat, lunch meat, bacon, ham, etc.

3. Consume less milk and milk products

4. Consume less fried foods

5. Consume less hydrogenated fats

6. Eat less refined flour products.

7. Eat less white sugar and simple sugars.

8. Eat less salt and salty foods, ie. Crackers, pretzels, chips, and pickled foods.

9. Consume fewer calories.

10. Consume less coffee and alcohol.

11. Smoke less or not at all.

12. Eat more fresh fruit.

13. Eat more fresh vegetables.

14. Eat more whole grain cereals, such as rice, whole wheat, oats, etc.

15. Eat more fiber foods – fruits, vegetables, grains.

16. Eat more fresh fish and poultry to replace red meats.

17. Eat more vegetable protein, such as nuts, seeds, and beans and the sprouts of these foods to replace animal proteins.

18. Drink more filtered or spring water.

19. Drink more (fresh) fruit and vegetable juices and herbal teas to replace coffee, black teas, soda pops, and other stimulating beverages.

20. Get more regular, preferable daily exercise with some aerobics.

21. Take better care of our air.

22. Keep our waters free of pollution.

(Staying Healthy with Nutrition, Elson M. Haas)

Appendix C – Multi-Vitamin Comparison

Jay Robb and Beach Body Multi-Vitamin Comparison

Jay Robb's Perfect Day Vitamin/Mineral EPA-DHA and Phytonutrient Formula

Vitamin A (67% beta-carotene, 33% palmitate)	15,000 IU	300%
Vitamin C (ascorbic acid)	500mg	833%
Vitamin D (50% D-2, 50% D-3)	800mg	200%
Vitamin E (d-alpha tocopherol)	200mg	667%
Vitamin K	50mcg	63%
Vitamin B-1 (thiamine mononitrate)	20mg	1333%
Vitamin B-2 (riboflavin)	30mg	1764%
Niacin-amide	30mg	150%
Vitamin B-6 (pyridoxine hydrochloride)	20mg	1000%
Folic Acid	400mcg	100%
Vitamin B-12 (cyanocobalamin)	200mcg	3333%
Biotin	75mcg	25%
Pantothenic Acid (Ca pantothenate)	25mg	250%
Calcium (80% citrate, 20% glycinate)	125mg	20%
Iodine (kelp)	150mcg	100%
Magnesium (80% oxide, 20% glycinate)	125mg	250%
Zinc (citrate)	10mg	67%
Selenium (L-selenomethionine)	50mccg	71%
Copper (citrate)	200mcg	100%
Chromium (citrate)	200mcg	167%
Molybdenum (sodium molybdate)	100mcg	133%

Potassium (citrate)	75mg	2%
Coral Calcium Powder (from Japan)	2000mg	
Marine Lipid Concentrate	2000mg	
(360mg EPA, 240mg DHA)		
Choline (bitartrate)	25mg	
Inositol (monophosphate)	30mg	
Boron (potassium borate)	3mg	
Silica (colloidal silica)	10mg	
Organic Horsetail	225mg	
Vanadium (vanadyl sulfate)	50mcg	
Fructooligosaccharides	200mg	
Calcium D-Glucarate	30mg	
Odorless Garlic (300mcg allicin)	100mg	
Green Tea Extract (10mg polyphenols)	30mg	
Glycyrrhizin (licorice root)	30mg	
Rosemary Extract	75mg	
Freeze-dried Broccoli	100mg	
Freeze-dried Tomatoes	100mg	
Freeze-dried Parsley	30mg	
Freeze-dried Celery	30mg	

BeachBody Multi-Vitamin

Vitamin A (acetate and beta-carotene)	10,000IU	200%
Vitamin C (calcium ascorbate)	500mg	833%
Vitamin D (cholecalciferol)	400IU	100%
Vitamin E (d-alpha tocopheryl succinate)	300IU	1000%
Thiamin (thiamine HCL)	75mg	5000%
Riboflavin	17mg	1000%
Niacin (niacin-amide)	100mg	500%
Vitamin B6 (pyridoxal 5 phosphate)	20mg	1000%
Folic Acid	800mcg	200%
Vitamin B12 (methylcobalamin)	600mcg	10,000%
Biotin	2mg	667%
Pantothenic Acid (Ca pantothenate)	50mg	500%
Calcium	400mg	40%
(carbonate, ascorbate, citrate, pantothenate)		
Iodine (potassium iodide)	150mcg	100%
Magnesium (mg oxide, mg chelate)	400mg	100%
Zinc (zinc citrate)	20mg	133%
Selenium (selenomethionine)	140mcg	200%
Copper (copper citrate)	2.5mg	125%
Manganese (Mg citrate)	10mg	500%
Chromium (polynicotinate)	240mcg	200%
Molybdenum (aspartate)	75mcg	100%
Boron (citrate)	2mg	
Vanadium (citrate)	40mcg	

Coenzyme Q10	10mg
Tocotrienols	2mg
N-Acetyl Cysteine	200mg
Alpha Lipoic Acid	25mg
Grape seed extract	25mg
Green Tea (Carnellia sinensis) leaf extract	25mg
Lutein	2mg
Bilberry extract (25% anthocyanidins)	10mg
Milk Thistle (80% silymarin)	50mg
Soy Isoflavones (standardized to 40%)	10mg
Ginkgo Biloba extract (24/6)	30mg
Vinpocetine	5mg
Beta Glucan (beta-1, 3-glucan)	20mg
Curcumin (95% cucuminoids)	100mg
Quercitin	100mg
Hesperidin	100mg
Trace Mineral Complex (72 minerals)	100mg
Arabinogalactan	20mg
Enzyme Delivery System	10mg

Appendix D - Auto-Immune Checklist

Autoimmune Symptoms: If you have these on a regular or continuing basis, you may have "Auto-Intoxication" which is an Auto-Immune disease where your body has too many toxins. You may want to consider doing a cleanse or a fast.

loss of muscle tone
memory loss
migraine
nausea
polyps
skin disorders
ulcers
yeast infections
high blood pressure
high cholesterol
immune problems
Infections
insomnia
intestinal obstruction
joint inflammation
confusion
depression
digestive problems
fainting
flatulence
fungal infections
gland or lymph problems
headache
abdominal pain
abdominal tenderness
acid reflux

low blood sugar levels
menstrual problems
nasal inflammation
parasitic infections
rectal bleeding
tissue degeneration
anemia
hemorrhoids
high blood sugar
hormonal imbalances
indigestion
inflammation
intestinal bleeding
allergies
joint pain
constipation
diarrhea
drowsiness
fatigue
bloating
excess gas
hair loss
abdominal cramping
abdominal swelling
abnormal growths
bacterial infection

Appendix E – Food Choices

Poor Food Choices

Toast	All Snack Foods
Waffle	Desserts
Bagel	White Rice
Pancakes	Soft Drinks
Milk	Bread
Processed Juice	Tortillas
Cookies	Ice Cream
Cereal	Candy
Pretzel	Pasta
Biscuit	Syrup
Beer	Donuts
Sandwich	French Fries
Cornstarch	Sugar
High Fructose Corn Syrup	

Better Food Choices

Eggs	Apple Cider Vinegar
Vegetables	Honey (raw)
Herbs	Real Cheese
Fresh Juice	Real Yogurt
Raw Nuts	Water
Olive Oil	Green Tea
Natural Sweeteners	Healthy Fats
Grass Fed Beef	Fish (no mercury)
Fresh Fruit (no pesticides)	

Appendix F - Glycemic Index

You want to try to eat the food that has a lower Glycemic number.

- **55 or less = Low (good)**

- **56- 69 = Medium**

- **70 or higher = High (bad)**

If you have blood sugar issues, you definitely want to try to stay with the slower-acting, good carbs. But, you can't look at the Glycemic Index in a Vacuum.   For example, a Snickers Bar has a Glycemic Index of 51, and Peanut M&M's are at 31. And a banana is 62. That doesn't mean you should eat candy in place of good food with a higher number.

The idea is that if you're going to buy cereal, compare cereal and choose one that has a lower number. If you're going to eat bread, choose one with a lower number. But from everything you've read to this point, you should know that you should be eating more fresh food and less processed food.

The following list comes from the Harvard Health Publications – Harvard Medical School

A - Glycemic index (glucose = 100)

B - Serving size (grams) (liquids are in mL)

C - Glycemic load per serving

BAKERY PRODUCTS AND BREADS

	A	B	C
Banana cake, made with sugar	47	60	14
Banana cake, made without sugar	55	60	12
Sponge cake, plain	46	63	17
Vanilla cake made from packet mix with vanilla frosting (Betty Crocker)	42	111	24
Apple, made with sugar	44	60	13
Apple, made without sugar	48	60	9
Waffles, Aunt Jemima (Quaker Oats)	76	35	10
Bagel, white, frozen	72	70	25
Baguette, white, plain	95	30	15
Coarse barley bread, 75-80% kernels, average	34	30	7
Hamburger bun	61	30	9
Kaiser roll	73	30	12
Pumpernickel bread	56	30	7
50% cracked wheat kernel bread	58	30	12
White wheat flour bread	71	30	10
Wonder bread, average	73	30	10
Whole wheat bread, average	71	30	9
100% Whole Grain bread	51	30	7
Pita bread, white	68	30	10
Corn tortilla	52	50	12
Wheat tortilla	30	50	8

BEVERAGES

	A	B	C
Coca Cola,	63	250	16
Fanta	68	250	23
Apple juice, unsweetened, average	44	250	30
Cranberry juice cocktail	68	250	24
Gatorade	78	250	12
Orange juice, unsweetened	50	250	12
Tomato juice, canned	38	250	4

BREAKFAST CEREALS AND RELATED PRODUCTS

	A	B	C
All-Bran, average	55	30	12
Coco Pops, average	77	30	20
Cornflakes, average	93	30	23
Cream of Wheat (Nabisco)	66	250	17
Cream of Wheat, Instant (Nabisco)	74	250	22
Grapenuts, average	75	30	16
Muesli, average	66	30	16
Oatmeal, average	55	250	13
Instant oatmeal, average	83	250	30
Puffed wheat, average	80	30	17
Raisin Bran (Kellogg's)	61	30	12
Special K (Kellogg's)	69	30	14

GRAINS

	A	B	C
Pearled barley, average	28	150	12
Sweet corn on the cob, average	60	150	20
Couscous, average	65	150	9
Quinoa	53	150	13
White rice, average	89	150	43
Quick cooking white basmati	67	150	28
Brown rice, average	50	150	16
Converted, white rice (Uncle Ben's)	38	150	14
Whole wheat kernels, average	30	50	11
Bulgur, average	48	150	12

COOKIES AND CRACKERS

	A	B	C
Graham crackers	74	25	14
Vanilla wafers	77	25	14
Shortbread	64	25	10
Rice cakes, average	82	25	17
Rye crisps, average	64	25	11
Soda crackers	74	25	12

DAIRY PRODUCTS AND ALTERNATIVES	A	B	C
Ice cream, regular	57	50	6
Ice cream, premium	38	50	3
Milk, full fat	41	250	5
Milk, skim	32	250	4
Reduced-fat yogurt w/ fruit, average	33	200	11

FRUITS			
Apple, average	39	120	6
Banana, ripe	62	120	16
Dates, dried	42	60	18
Grapefruit	25	120	3
Grapes, average	59	120	11
Orange, average	40	120	4
Peach, average	42	120	5
Peach, canned in light syrup	40	120	5
Pear, average	38	120	4
Pear, canned in pear juice	43	120	5
Prunes, pitted	29	60	10
Raisins	64	60	28
Watermelon	72	120	4

BEANS AND NUTS

	A	B	C
Baked beans, average	40	150	6
Blackeyed peas, average	33	150	10
Black beans	30	150	7
Chickpeas, average	10	150	3
Chickpeas, canned in brine	38	150	9
Navy beans, average	31	150	9
Kidney beans, average	29	150	7
Lentils, average	29	150	5
Soy beans, average	15	150	1
Cashews, salted	27	50	3
Peanuts, average	7	50	0

PASTA and NOODLES

	A	B	C
Fettuccine, average	32	180	15
Macaroni, average	47	180	23
Macaroni and Cheese (Kraft)	64	180	32
Spaghetti, white, boiled, average	46	180	22
Spaghetti, white, average	58	180	26
Spaghetti, wholemeal, boiled, average	42	180	17

SNACK FOODS

	A	B	C
Corn chips, plain, salted, average	42	50	11
Fruit Roll-Ups	99	30	24
M & M's, peanut	33	30	6
Microwave popcorn, plain, average	55	20	6
Potato chips, average	51	50	12
Pretzels, oven-baked	83	30	16
Snickers Bar	51	60	18

VEGETABLES

	A	B	C
Green peas, average	51	80	4
Carrots, average	35	80	2
Parsnips	52	80	4
Baked russet potato, average	111	150	33
Boiled white potato, average	82	150	21
Instant mashed potato, average	87	150	17
Sweet potato, average	70	150	22
Yam, average	54	150	20

MISCELLANEOUS

	A	B	C
Hummus (chickpea salad dip)	6	30	0
Chicken nuggets, frozen,	46	100	7
Honey, average	61	25	12

211

Appendix G - Food Combining

Some people believe that your body's digestive system works better by combining food in certain ways. This, they claim, not only helps digestion, but by extension, your overall health. Proper food combining can:

- Improve digestion and absorption

- Help balance pH

- Improve energy levels

There are 4 general rules for food combining:

1. Fruits should be eaten alone or with other fruits

    a. Acid fruit should not be combined with sweet fruits

    b. Melons should be eaten alone

2. Proteins and starches should not be eaten together

3. Eat protein with vegetables, or starch and vegetables

4. Don't eat more than one protein food per meal

There are many types of Food Combining Charts that may be useful for you. I suggest you give it a try and see how it affects you. It works for a lot of people.

There are some good pictographs on food combining online. Try going to www.bing.com/images and type in Food Combining.

Appendix H - Running the Numbers

1 lb = 3500 calories

If you reduce your caloric intake by 200 calories per day and

Increase your expenditure by 300 calories per day...

Your net caloric change is 500 calories per day x 7 days is 3500 calories (or 1 lb) per week

Calculating your caloric intake and grams needed

First, calculate the number of calories you need or want for your health goal.

Second, apply your Carb, Protein, Fat ratio. Count the calories. Translate to grams.

Example:

To lose 20lbs, I want to eat 1800 calories per day (this number can be different depending on the individual.)

My Carb:Protein:Fat ratio is 40:30:30

1800 calories x 40% = 720 carb calories / 4 grams/cal = 180 grams

1800 calories x 30% = 540 protein calories / 4 grams/cal = 135 grams

1800 calories x 30% = 540 fat calories / 9 grams/cal = 60 grams

If you want to do the 20:45:35 (carb:protein:fat):

1800 calories x 20% = 360 carb calories / 4 grams/cal = 90 grams

1800 calories x 45% = 810 protein calories / 4 grams/cal = 202 grams

1800 calories x 35% = 630 fat calories / 9 grams/cal = 70 grams

YOU:

_____ calories X _____% carb calories / 4 grams/cal =

_____ grams

_____ calories x _____% protein calories /4 grams/cal =

_____ grams

_____ calories x _____% fat calories / 9 grams/cal =

_____ grams

Appendix I - Important Food Facts

Top 10 Hydrating Foods

Cucumber – 96% water

Watermelon – 96% water

Pineapple – 95% water

Tomato – 94% water

Blueberries – 95% water

Celery – 95% water

Cantaloupe – 92% water

Grapefruit – 90% water

Pair – 89% water

(www.HealingPowerHour.com)

Top 8 Nutrient Dense Foods

Spirulina – has more antioxidants than any other food. Lots of protein and minerals

Kale – Abundance of vitamins, minerals, amino acids, fiber, and antioxidants

Hemp Seeds – Contains vitamins, minerals, amino acids, antioxidants, fatty acids, fiber, and protein

Chocolate – Contains vitamins, minerals, and antioxidants

Broccoli – Excellent for digestion and may decrease your risk of cancer

Spinach – Contains protein, fiber, and antioxidants

Chia Seeds – Contains protein, fiber, and omega fats

Berries – Contains vitamins, minerals, and antioxidants

(www.juicewithdrew.com)

Metabolic Boosting Foods

Almonds	Apples	Asparagus	Beans
Berries	Broccoli	Cabbage	Carrots
Celery	Cucumber	Curry	Eggs
Garlic	Grapefruit	Lemons	Limes
Oats	Oranges	Spinach	Tomatoes
Peanut Butter	Spicy Peppers		

(don't-feed-alex.tumblr.com)

Simple Food Changes

Change:	To:
White Sugar	Brown Sugar
Artificial Sweetener	Stevia
Milk (from cows)	Coconut/Almond Milk
Butter	Coconut Oil
White Rice	Brown Rice
White Potatoes	Sweet Potatoes
Canola Oil	Coconut or Olive Oil
Table Salt	Sea Salt
Salad Dressing	Oil and Vinegar
Pre-packaged Juice	Fresh Juice

Appendix J - Grocery Shopping List

Vegetables

Alfalfa sprouts	Green beans
Asparagus	Kale
Beets	Mushrooms
Bell peppers	Mustard greens
Broccoli	Onions
Brussel sprouts	Parsnips
Cabbage	Peas
Cauliflower	Pumpkin
Celery	Spinach
Collard greens	Squash
Cucumbers	Sweet Potatoes
Eggplant	Swiss chard
Garlic	Tomatoes

Fruit

Apples	Limes
Apricots	Mango
Bananas	Nectarines
Blueberries	Oranges
Cantaloupe	Papaya
Cherries	Peaches
Cranberries	Pears
Dates	Pineapple
Grapefruit	Plums
Grapes	Pomegranates
Honeydew	Prunes
Kiwi	Raisins
Lemons	Raspberries

Grocery Shopping List

Grains/Legumes

Barley	Quinoa
Brown rice	Rye
Buckwheat	Spelt
Millet	Whole wheat
Oats	Beans

Protein

Cod	Lamb
Halibut	Venison
Salmon	Protein powder
Sardines	Eggs
Tuna	Tofu
Grass-fed beef	Free range chicken

Fats

Almonds	Olives
Almond Butter	Peanut butter (real)
Avocado	Pumpkin seeds
Cashews	Sesame seeds
Coconut Oil	Sunflower seeds
Flaxseeds	Walnuts

Grocery Shopping List

Herbs/Spices

Basil	Ginger
Cayenne pepper	Mint
Cilantro	Mustard seeds
Cinnamon	Oregano
Cumin	Rosemary
Dill	Turmeric

Natural Sweeteners

Agave	Pure maple syrup
Blackstrap Molasses	Xylitol
Raw Honey	Stevia

Appendix K – Your Home Gym List

You don't have to buy everything at once. You can buy one or two pieces at a time. Keep track. Check them off one at a time, and write down the date.

Home Gym Checklist			Bought (X)	Date
1	Yoga Mat	$ 20.00		
1	Large Exercise Ball	$ 20.00		
1	Jump Rope	$ 10.00		
3	Resistance Bands	$ 30.00		
1	Bosu Ball	$ 125.00		
1	Medicine Ball	$ 30.00		
1	Set of Dumbells	$ 300.00		
	3lb			
	5lb			
	10lb			
	15lb			
	20lb			
	30lb			
	40lb			
1	Weight Bench	$ 175.00		
1	Heart Rate Monitor	$ 75.00		
	Total	$ 785.00		

Appendix L - Reading List

Reading List	Author
Curing The Cause & Preventing Disease	Dr. Steven Ross, DC, FASBE, DAAPM
Herbs of the Bible	James A. Duke, PhD
Fitness: The Complete Guide	Frederick C. Hatfield, PhD
Nutrition Amanac	Dunne
Human Functional Anatomy	Schlossberg & Zuidema
The Advanced Guide to Longevity Medicine	Ghen
The Cleanse Cookbook	Christine Dreher
Diet and Nutrition	Rudolph Ballentine, MD
Staying Healthy with Nutrtion	Elson Hass, MD
Glutathione: The Ultimate Antioxidant	Alan H. Pressman, DC, PhD
The Wellness Revolution	Pilzer
Fresh Vegetables & Fruit Juices	Dr. N. W. Walker
The Acid-Alkaline Balance Diet	Klimet
The Healing Revolution	Dr. Frank King
Cleanse & Purify Thyself	Richard Anderson, ND, NMD
Eat Live, Be Alive	Dr. Moira Casey, DC
Wheat Belly	William Davis, MD
Sugar Busters	H. Leighton Steward
The Complete Self-Care Guide to Holistic Medicine	Ivker, Anderson, & Trivieri
Fasting and Eating for Health	Joel Fuhrman, MD
Putting It All Together: The New Orthomolecular Nutrition	Hoffer & Walker
Miracle of Fasting	Patricia Bragg
Fat Buring Diet	Jay Robb
Homeopathic Medicine at Home	Panos & Heimlich
The Doctor's Heart Cure	Al Sears, MD
Complete Physiquie - A Program of E.N.E.R.G.Y.	Infiinity
Nutribase Complete Book of Food Counts	Dr. Art Ulene
Body Reflexology	Carter
Food - Your Miracle Medicine	Jean Carper
The Ultimate Healing System	Dr. Donald J. Lepore, ND
Solved: The Riddle of Illness	Langer & Scheer
New Herb Bible	Earl Mindell, R.Ph, PhD
Food as Medicine	Dharma Singh Khalsa, MD
Naturopathy for the 21st Century	Robert J. Thiel, PhD
Enymes: The Key to Health	Loomis
Prescription for Nutritional Healing	Phyllis A. Balch, CNC
The Carbohydrate Addict's Diet	R. Rachael F. Heller & Dr. Richard F. Heller
The Juicing Book	Stephen Blauer
The Nutritional Cost of Prescription Drugs	Ross Pelton & James B. LaValle, R.Ph

Appendix M - Resources

Schools

Natural Healing Institute
515 Encinitas Blvd. #201
Encinitas, CA 92024
760-943-8485

A2Z Health
2955 N. Moorpark Rd.
Thousand Oaks, CA 91360
805-241-4194

Websites
www.naturalnews.com
www.foodmatters.tv
www.jayrobb.com
www.nhicollege.com
www.a2zhealth.com
www.ulti-health.com
www.billystixworkout.com
www.profhudson.com
www.hoomanainstitute.com
www.ajjf.org

Good Quality Products
Metagenics
Douglas Laboratories
Biotics
SafeCareRx
Arise and Shine
Beach Body
Primal Force
Jay Robb

www.ingramcontent.com/pod-product-compliance
Lightning Source LLC
Chambersburg PA
CBHW070638290526
45790CB00001B/132